CLINICAL DECISION MAKING

Case Studies in Pharmacology

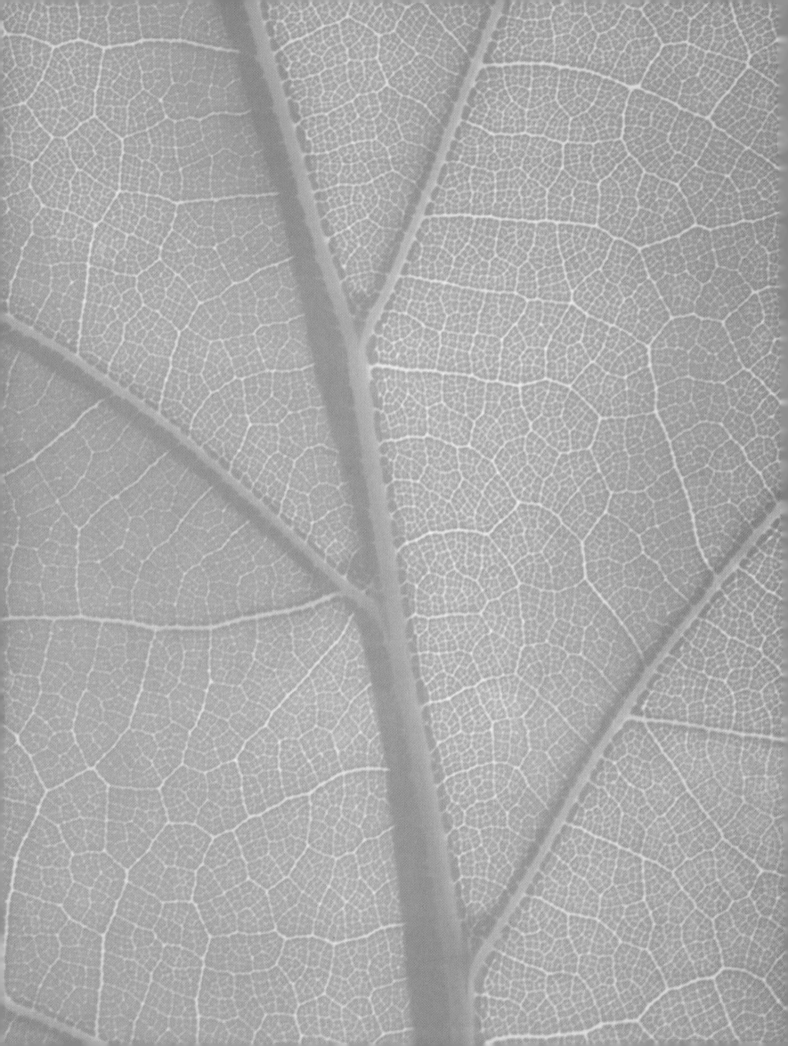

CLINICAL DECISION MAKING

Case Studies
in Pharmacology

Hyacinth C. Martin
BSN, MA, MSEd, MPS, RNBC

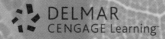

DELMAR
CENGAGE Learning

Australia • Brazil • Japan • Korea • Mexico • Singapore • Spain • United Kingdom • United States

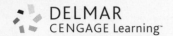

Clinical Decision Making: Case Studies in Pharmacology
Hyacinth C. Martin

Vice President, Health Care Business Unit:
  William Brottmiller

Director of Learning Solutions: Matthew Kane

Acquisitions Editor: Maureen Rosener

Product Manager: Elizabeth Howe

Editorial Assistant: Chelsey Iaquinta

Marketing Director: Jennifer McAvey

Marketing Manager: Michele McTighe

Marketing Coordinator: Danielle Pacella

Production Director: Carolyn Miller

Content Project Manager: Jessica McNavich

For product information and technology assistance, contact us at
Cengage Learning Customer & Sales Support, 1-800-354-9706

For permission to use material from this text or product,
submit all requests online at **www.cengage.com/permissions**
Further permissions questions can be emailed to
permissionrequest@cengage.com

Library of Congress Control Number: 2006007600

ISBN-13: 978-1-4018-3521-7

ISBN-10: 1-4018-3521-X

Delmar
Executive Woods
5 Maxwell Drive
Clifton Park, NY 12065
USA

Cengage Learning is a leading provider of customized learning solutions with office locations around the globe, including Singapore, the United Kingdom, Australia, Mexico, Brazil, and Japan. Locate your local office at **www.cengage.com/global**

Cengage Learning products are represented in Canada by Nelson Education, Ltd.

To learn more about Delmar, visit **www.cengage.com/delmar**

Purchase any of our products at your local bookstore or at our preferred online store **www.cengagebrain.com**

Notice to the Reader
Publisher does not warrant or guarantee any of the products described herein or perform any independent analysis in connection with any of the product information contained herein. Publisher does not assume, and expressly disclaims, any obligation to obtain and include information other than that provided to it by the manufacturer. The reader is expressly warned to consider and adopt all safety precautions that might be indicated by the activities described herein and to avoid all potential hazards. By following the instructions contained herein, the reader willingly assumes all risks in connection with such instructions. The publisher makes no representations or warranties of any kind, including but not limited to, the warranties of fitness for particular purpose or merchantability, nor are any such representations implied with respect to the material set forth herein, and the publisher takes no responsibility with respect to such material. The publisher shall not be liable for any special, consequential, or exemplary damages resulting, in whole or part, from the readers' use of, or reliance upon, this material.

Printed in the United States of America
3 4 5 6 7 16 15 14 13 12

Contents

Part 4 The Nervous System 119

Part 5 The Endocrine System 135

Part 6 The Musculoskeletal and Reproductive Systems 155

Reviewers

Mary Beth Kiefner, RN, MS
Nursing Program Director
Nursing Faculty, Illinois Central College
East Peoria, Illinois

Joan Piper Mader, RN, MSN
Associate Professor or Nursing
College of the Mainland
Texas City, Texas

Darla R. Ura, MA, RN, APRN, BC
Clinical Associate Professor
Department of Adult and Elder Health Nursing
School of Nursing, Emory University
Atlanta, Georgia

Mari A. Smith, DSN, RN, CCRN
Professor
School of Nursing, Middle Tennessee State University
Murfreesboro, Tennessee

Preface

Delmar's Case Study Series was created to encourage nurses to bridge the gap between content knowledge and clinical application. The products within the series represent the most innovative and comprehensive approach to nursing case studies ever developed. Each title has been authored by experienced nurse educators and clinicians who understand the complexity of nursing practice as well as the challenges of teaching and learning. All of the cases are based on real-life clinical scenarios and demand thought and "action" from the nurse. Each case brings the user into the clinical setting and invites her to utilize the nursing process while considering all of the variables that influence the client's condition and the care to be provided. Each case also represents a unique set of variables to offer a breadth of learning experiences and to capture the reality of nursing practice. To gauge the progression of a user's knowledge and critical thinking ability, the cases have been categorized by difficulty level. Every section begins with basic cases and proceeds to more advanced scenarios, thereby presenting opportunities for learning and practice for both students and professionals.

All of the cases have been expert reviewed to ensure that as many variables as possible are represented in a truly realistic manner and that each case reflects consistency with realities of modern nursing practice.

How to Use This Book

Every case begins with a table of variables that are encountered in practice, and that must be understood by the nurse in order to provide appropriate care to the client. Categories of variables include age, gender, setting, culture, ethnicity, cultural considerations, preexisting conditions, coexisting conditions, communication considerations, disability considerations, socioeconomic considerations, spiritual considerations, pharmacological considerations, psychosocial considerations, legal considerations, ethical considerations, alternative therapy, prioritization considerations, and delegation considerations. If a case involves a variable that is considered to have a significant impact on care, the specific variable is included in the table. This allows the user an "at-a-glance" view of the issues that will need to be considered to provide care to the client in the scenario. The table of variables is followed by a presentation of the case, including the history of the client, current condition, clinical setting, and professionals involved. A series of questions follows each case that ask the user to consider how she would handle the issues presented within the scenario.

Organization

Cases are grouped according to body system. Within each part, cases are organized by difficulty level from easy, to moderate, to difficult. This classification is somewhat subjective, but it is based upon a developed standard. In general, difficulty level has been determined by the number of variables that impact the case and the complexity of the client's condition. Colored tabs are used to allow the user to distinguish the difficulty levels more easily. A comprehensive table of variables is also provided for reference, to allow the user to quickly select cases containing a particular variable of care.

While every effort has been made to group cases into the most applicable body system, the scope of many of the cases may include more than one body system. In such instances, the case will still only appear in the section for one of the body systems addressed. The cases are fictitious; however, they are based on actual problems and/or situations the nurse will encounter. Any resemblance to actual cases or individuals is coincidental.

Praise for Delmar's Case Study Series

"[This text's] strength is the large variety of case studies – it seemed to be all inclusive. Another strength is the extensiveness built into each case study. You can almost see this person as they enter the ED because of the descriptions that are given."

—MARY BETH KIEFNER, RN, MS
Nursing Program Director/Nursing Faculty,
Illinois Central College

"The cases . . . reflect the complexity of nursing practice. They are an excellent way to refine critical thinking skills."

—DARLA R. URA, MA, RN, APRN, BC
Clinical Associate Professor, Department of
Adult and Elder Health Nursing, School of
Nursing, Emory University

"This text does an excellent job of reflecting the complexity of nursing practice."

—VICKI NEES, RNC, MSN, APRN-BC
Associate Professor,
Ivy Tech State College

". . . the case studies are very comprehensive and allow the undergraduate student an opportunity to apply knowledge gained in the classroom to a potentially real clinical situation."

—TAMELLA LIVENGOOD, APRN, BC, MSN, FNP
Nursing Faculty,
Northwestern Michigan College

"These cases and how you have approached them definitely stimulate the students to use critical-thinking skills. I thought the questions asked really pushed the students to think deeply and thoroughly."

—JOANNE SOLCHANY, PHD, ARNP, RN, CS
Assistant Professor,
Family & Child Nursing,
University of Washington, Seattle

"The use of case studies is pedagogically sound and very appealing to students and instructors. I think that some instructors avoid them because of the challenge of case development. You have provided the material for them."

—NANCY L. OLDENBURG, RN, MS, CPNP
Clinical Instructor,
Northern Illinois University

"[The author] has done an excellent job of assisting students to engage in critical thinking. I am very impressed with the cases, questions and content. I rarely ask that students buy more than one . . . book . . . but, in this instance, I can't wait until this book is published."

—DEBORAH J. PERSELL, MSN, RN, CPNP
Assistant Professor,
Arkansas State University

"This is a groundbreaking book. . . . This book should be a required text for all undergraduate and graduate nursing programs and should be well-received by faculty."

—JANE H. BARNSTEINER, PhD, RN, FAAN
Professor of Pediatric Nursing,
University of Pennsylvania School of Nursing

About the Author

Hyacinth C. Martin was first influenced by her elementary school teacher in choosing nursing as a career. However, the major influential persons in her choice of nursing as a career were nurses who wore white uniforms, white shoes, including nursing hats, and who seemed to have generated the highest respect from those they came in contact with. Hyacinth's nursing career includes staff nurse experiences on medical-surgical units, head nurse/nurse manager for medical-surgical units and critical-care units, administrative nursing supervisor, community nursing, and administrative nursing supervisor in long-term care agencies. Her academic experiences include teaching theory and clinical in a Licensed Practical Nursing program, a Baccalaureate Degree Program and at present in an Associate Degree program. In 1999, Hyacinth was a guest speaker on WMBC-TV (Channel 63, Newton, NJ), discussing issues pertaining to multiculturalism, with a focus on multicultural marriage and its effects on the family.

Publications include two articles for a nursing journal, one manuscript for Continuing Medical Education Resource, and part of a chapter on the endocrine system, published by Delmar, Cengage Learning. She has also reviewed a chapter in *Pharmacology for Nursing Care*, Richard A. Lehne (5th ed.), and revised *PowerPoint for Pharmacology for Nursing Care* (6th ed.) and an instructor's manual. She was a contributor for *Gerontological Nursing Textbook* (2006), P. A. Tabloski.

Her contributions to education include recent presentations: "Pulmonary Tuberculosis: Controlling the Transmission of the Disease," at PACE University Conference; "Civic Society, Environmental Responsibility, & Sustainable Development in the United States & Brazil," presented at the Manhattan Veteran's Hospital Medical Center Conference, New York; and "The Effective Use of Unfractionated and Fractionated Heparin Therapy to Patients at Risk for Thrombus Formation" and "Nurse's Nurturing Nurses," presented at Lincoln Hospital Medical Center, New York.

Achievements

Hyacinth Martin was recognized in Who's Who Among American Teachers for four successive years. A current recipient of a PSC-CUNY Grant for research on Gender and Career Choice in Nursing, she is a full-time tenured professor in the nursing program at Borough of Manhattan Community College/The City University of New York. Her passion in teaching is to assist in the success of students who enroll in the nursing program at Borough of Manhattan Community College.

Hyacinth's other contributions (along with her husband's) to the welfare of others include adopting a basic school in one of the West Indian islands, and sponsoring a nursing student in Davao City, Philippines. Hyacinth earned a BSN degree and a Master's Degree in Career Guidance and Counseling from Lehman College, a Master's Degree in Nursing Administration from Columbia University, and a Master's Degree in Urban Education/Theology from NYACK College, New York. She is currently pursuing a doctoral degree in theology.

Acknowledgments

I want to express my sincere thanks to Elizabeth Howe, Product Manager, for the professional manner in which she communicated with me both verbally and by e-mail. I also want to thank the entire editorial staff at Delmar, Cengage Learning for guidance in writing this text. I wish to record my thanks to the accuracy reviewer, Bonita E. Broyles, RN, BSN, EdD. Your excellent guidance removed much of the stress that writing the text generated. A special thanks to Reverend Florentina Lapsey and Professor Louise Green for their constant prayers as I pursued the task of research and writing the text. I am grateful to Dr. David Ephraim for his encouragement and the many hours spent making sure computers and laptops were functioning, and lost content restored. Lastly, thank you, Professor Boyle-Egland for that special moment of support as the text was entering its final stage.

This book is dedicated to:

My granddaughter, Nardia – May you also become the author of many books.

My husband, Frederick, a retired registered nurse himself, in recognition of all that I owe him for his patience and understanding as he took on the responsibility of most of the household chores to enable me to accomplish this goal. It is my hope and prayer that this modest work will assist nursing students to better understand the content of medical-surgical nursing and, in so doing, help them to appreciate more of the incredible writings of nurse authors.

Hyacinth C. Martin

Comprehensive Table of Variables

Case Study	Gender	Age	Setting	Ethnicity/Culture	Preexisting Conditions	Coexisting Conditions	Lifestyle	Communication	Disability	Socioeconomic	Spiritual/Religious	Pharmacologic	Psychosocial	Legal	Ethical	Alternative Therapy	Prioritization	Delegation
Part One: The Digestive and Urinary Systems																		
1	M	64	Hospital	White American	×		×				×	×	×			×	×	×
2	M	34	Clinic	Japanese/Asian			×	×			×	×	×			×	×	×
3	M	52	"Outpatient, urology clinic"	Mexican American	×	×	×			×	×	×	×	×	×	×	×	×
4	F	35	Hospital	White American		×	×					×	×			×	×	×
5	F	60	Hospital	Black American	×		×				×	×	×		×		×	×
6	M	38	Hospital	Black American/West Indian			×				×	×	×				×	×
7	M	70	Hospital	Black American		×	×				×	×	×		×	×	×	×
8	M	64	Hospital	White American			×				×	×	×				×	×
Part Two: The Respiratory and Immune Systems																		
1	M	76	Skilled nursing facility	White American		×	×		×	×	×	×	×	×			×	×
2	F	32	"Clinic, tertiary care center of medical center"	Black/South African			×	×			×	×	×	×	×	×	×	×
3	M	50	Hospital	White American	×	×	×			×	×	×	×	×		×	×	×
4	M	55	Hospital	Black American	×	×	×		×	×	×	×	×		×	×	×	×
5	F	60	Hospital	African/Nigerian	×	×	×		×		×	×	×	×		×	×	×
6	M	62	Hospital	Italian/American			×				×	×	×				×	×
7	M	42	Hospital	Black American	×	×	×	×		×	×	×	×	×		×	×	×
8	M	40	Hospital	Hispanic American	×	×	×				×	×	×	×		×	×	×
Part Three: The Cardiovascular and Lymphatic Systems																		
1	M	65	ER	Black American	×	×	×				×	×	×			×	×	×
2	F	68	Outpatient	White American	×	×	×		×	×	×	×	×	×		×	×	×
3	M	78	Hospital	Black American	×	×	×				×	×	×			×	×	×
4	F	56	Hospital	Black American	×	×	×				×	×	×			×	×	×
5	F	60	Hospital	Hispanic American	×	×	×				×	×	×		×	×	×	×
6	M	66	Hospital	White American	×	×	×				×	×	×			×	×	×

7	M	56	Hospital	Hispanic American
8	M	54	Outpatient	White American
9	F	64	Hospital	Black American
10	M	60	Hospital clinic	White Portuguese
11	M	72		White American
12	M	72	Adult home/hospital	Black American/West Indian

Part Four: The Nervous System

1	M	30	Clinic	Hispanic American
2	F	38	Hospital	White American
3	F	24	ER	Black American/West Indian
4	F	42	Hospital	mixed race

Part Five: The Endocrine System

1	F	30	Office	Black American/West Indian
2	F	42	Hospital	Native American/Argentina
3	M	20	Hospital	Hispanic American
4	F	50	Hospital	White American
5	F	56	Office	Black American/West Indian

Part Six: The Musculoskeletal and Reproductive Systems

1	F	25	Clinic	Native American
2	M	32	Hospital	Black American/West Indian
3	M	64	Hospital	White American
4	F	58	Clinic	Black American
5	F	40	Hospital	Black American
6	M	30	Hospital	Black American

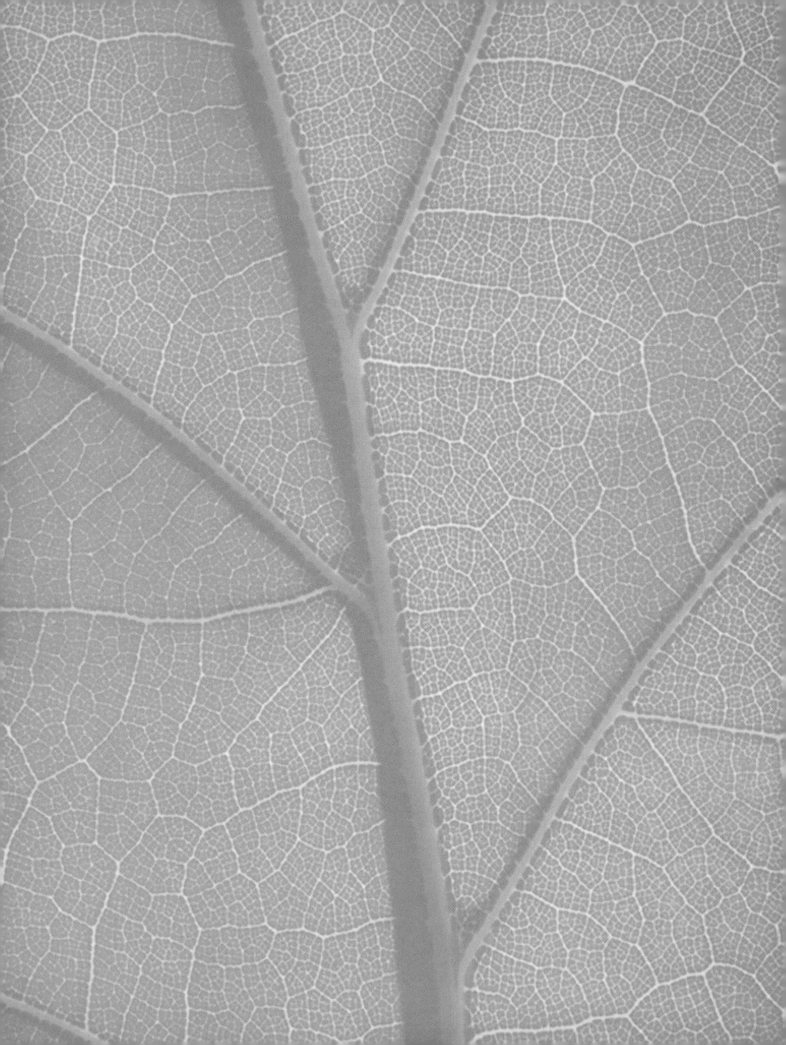

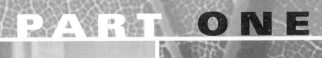

PART ONE

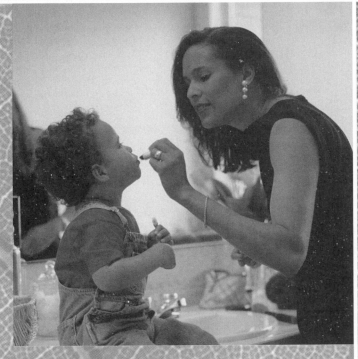

The Digestive and Urinary Systems

Cyanocobalamin (Vitamin B_{12} Deficiency Anemia, Pernicious Anemia)

GENDER

M

AGE

64

SETTING

- Hospital

ETHNICITY/CULTURE

- White

PREEXISTING CONDITIONS

- Zollinger-Ellison syndrome

COEXISTING CONDITIONS

- Total gastrectomy

LIFESTYLE

- Retired

COMMUNICATION

DISABILITY

SOCIOECONOMIC STATUS

- Middle

SPIRITUAL/RELIGIOUS

- Catholic

PHARMACOLOGIC

- Vitamin B_{12}
- Folic acid (Apo-Folic)

PSYCHOSOCIAL

- Periods of irritability and depression

LEGAL

ETHICAL

ALTERNATIVE THERAPY

- Clams
- Frankfurters
- Red beans

PRIORITIZATION

- Monitor for signs of alteration in cognition or irritability

DELEGATION

- RN
- Client education

THE DIGESTIVE AND URINARY SYSTEMS

Level of difficulty: Easy

Overview: This case involves a thorough assessment of the past medical and surgical history. The nurse must observe the client for signs of impaired memory or irritability during the assessment.

Client Profile

Mr. L is a 64-year-old client who had a total gastrectomy of the small and large bowel resection including the ileum two years ago. Mr. L is referred to the hospital inpatient clinic by his primary health care provider for further evaluation after a routine annual examination.

Case Study

During the initial interview, Mr. L complains of having had anorexia, nausea, vomiting, and abdominal pain for the past two days. Physical assessment findings include paresthesia of the hands and feet, reduced vibratory and position senses, ataxia, and muscle weakness. Assessment data on his daily nutritional intake includes frankfurters, brewer's yeast, clams, dried beans, and carrots. Vital signs taken by the nursing assistant are:

> Blood pressure: 120/78
>
> Pulse: 78
>
> Respirations: 18
>
> Temperature: 98.4° F

Tentative diagnosis of pernicious anemia is made and the health care provider prescribes serum laboratory data: hematocrit, hemoglobin, methylmalonic acid and homocysteine level, platelet count, red blood cell count, folic acid level, and peripheral blood smear. Mr. L is to return to the clinic in two days for a follow-up on the results of the laboratory data, confirmation of the diagnosis, and prescription as required. Mr. L returns to the clinic as scheduled. His laboratory results are:

> Hematocrit (Hct): 38%
>
> Hemoglobin (Hgb): 16 g/dL
>
> Methylmalonic acid and homocysteine levels: elevated
>
> Platelet count: 200,000/mm^3
>
> Red blood cell (RBC) count: 2,500,000/mm^3
>
> Folic acid: 3 ng/mL

Also, the peripheral blood smear shows oval, macrocytic, and hyperchromic RBCs. The health care provider reviews the data, and a diagnosis of pernicious anemia is confirmed.

The following are prescribed:
- Cyanocobalamin (vitamin B$_{12}$) 2,000 mcg PO per day for two weeks, then 1,000 mcg PO per day
- Folic acid (Apo-Folic) 0.4 mg PO daily

Questions

1. Explain the pathophysiology of vitamin B_{12} deficiency and its relationship to pernicious anemia.

2. Why is vitamin B_{12} anemia called megaloblastic anemia?

3. Discuss classic manifestations of vitamin B_{12} deficiency anemia a nurse should expect to observe during assessment of this client.

4. Discuss the specific relationship of erythrocytes (RBCs) and vitamin B_{12} deficiency and nursing management.

5. Discuss common nursing diagnoses for vitamin B_{12} deficiency anemia.

6. What are the purposes for the prescribed medications?

7. What are the most common adverse reactions, drug-to-drug, drug-to-food/herbal interactions of cyanocobalamin (vitamin B_{12})?

8. Discuss factors that may inhibit folic acid absorption.

9. Discuss client education for vitamin B_{12} deficiency anemia.

10. Discuss nursing implications for clients with vitamin B_{12} deficiency anemia.

Renal Calculi

GENDER

M

AGE

34

SETTING

- Clinic

ETHNICITY/CULTURE

- Japanese/Asian

PREEXISTING CONDITIONS

COEXISTING CONDITIONS

LIFESTYLE

- Employed for the last four years as a computer analyst for a U.S. company

COMMUNICATION

- English as a second language

DISABILITY

SOCIOECONOMIC STATUS

- Upper

SPIRITUAL/RELIGIOUS

- Shinto

PHARMACOLOGIC

- Morphine sulfate (Duramorph)
- Oxybutynin chloride (Ditropan)
- Hydrochlorothiazide (HydroDIURIL)

PSYCHOSOCIAL

- Fear
- Pain
- Anxiety

LEGAL

ETHICAL

ALTERNATIVE THERAPY

- Imagery
- Relaxation techniques

PRIORITIZATION

- Pain management
- Prevent kidney damage

DELEGATION

- RN
- Client education

THE DIGESTIVE AND URINARY SYSTEMS

Level of difficulty: Easy

Overview: This case involves pain management as well as questioning the client about personal or family history of urologic stones, obtaining a diet history, including fluid intake patterns. If the client has a history of stone formation, it should be determined if chemical analysis of the stone(s) was performed in the past and what the preventive measures were.

Client Profile

Mr. J is a 34-year-old male who arrives at the emergency department (ED) of a busy urban hospital accompanied by his brother, who drove Mr. J from his office to the ED. Mr. J is 5′6″ and weighs 134 pounds.

Case Study

On arrival, Mr. J reports an "unbearable" pain that is intermittent in nature. He describes the pain as more intense while he was walking to his brother's car. Mr. J also reports that the pain began insidiously, one day ago, and he noticed it while working at his desk. He said that, later that day, he felt nauseated and was diaphoretic. He tried to take some fluids but the nausea would not subside, which decreased his fluid intake. Later that night, he felt warm, but did not know what his temperature was. Upon awakening in the morning, the pain had decreased much. However, when he urinated, the amount was small, and the color was pink-red. He prepared and left for work, trying to avoid the discomfort. While preparing a report for presentation at a luncheon meeting, he felt a pain that radiated from his left side to his abdomen. The pain was severe for about one minute. He informed his brother, who works in an adjoining building, and the brother transported him to the ED. Mr. J denies previous episodes of this type of pain. He reports no past or current medication history. Social history includes racquetball on weekends, occasional games of tennis, and he enjoys drinking white wine with the evening meal, which usually includes rhubarb and wheat germ. He is triaged by a nurse. His vital signs are:

Blood pressure: 130/82

Pulse: 94 and regular

Respirations: 18

Temperature: 101.0° F

He is seen by the ED health care provider, who does a history and physical, then orders a stat dose of morphine sulfate 5 mg/SQ. An intravenous line with dextrose 5% and 0.45 sodium chloride at 100 mL/hr is initiated. A computed tomography (CT) scan is done and calcium oxalate stones are identified in the left kidney calyx. A urine dipstick test is positive for hematuria, and urinalysis reveals red blood cells (RBCs) in the urine. There is no turbidity or odor from the urine specimen. Mr. J's laboratory results are:

Serum calcium: 10.5 mg/dL

Serum phosphate: 5 mg/dL

Serum uric acid: 9 mg/dL

Urine uric acid: 800 mg/24 hr

Urine calcium: 260 mg/24 hr

Urine phosphate: 1.3 g/24 hr

Urine specific gravity: 1.026

After the health care provider reviews the laboratory data and diagnostic results, a diagnosis of renal calculi is confirmed. Mr. J's pain has subsided and he denies feeling nauseated. He has voided 100 mL of dusky-colored urine with trace elements of blood. The urine is strained and there is one visible stone. A sample of the urine is sent to the lab for microscopic analysis. Mr. J's vital signs are:

Blood pressure: 110/70

Pulse: 78 and regular

Respirations: 14

Temperature: 98.4° F

Mr. J will be discharged in the late evening. Mr. J is to return to his primary health care provider for follow-up care in two weeks.

The following are prescribed:

- Morphine sulfate (Astromorph PF) 1–2 mg IV q1–2h
- Oxybutynin chloride (Ditropan) 5 mg PO two times per day, today only
- Hydrochlorothiazide (HydroDIURIL) 50 mg PO two times per day
- IV D 5.45% NS at 100 mL/hr until 5:00 PM today and encourage fluid intake of two to three liters today
- Accurate intake and output, and strain all urine
- Discharge after 5:00 PM with follow-up appointment in two weeks

Questions

1. Discuss factors that contribute to urolithiasis.

2. Discuss the most common types of kidney stones.

3. Discuss common manifestations of urolithiasis.

4. Discuss common complications of urolithiasis.

5. What are the purposes for the prescribed orders?

6. What are the most common adverse reactions, drug-to-drug, drug-to-food/herbal interactions of the prescribed medications?

7. Discuss other diagnostic tests used to identify urolithiasis.

8. Discuss endourologic procedures used to remove or crush urolithiasis.

9. Discuss the difference between a ureterolithotomy and a pyelolithotomy.

10. Discuss client education for urolithiasis.

Stage IIC Cancer of the Prostate

GENDER

Male

AGE

52

SETTING

- Urology outpatient clinic of a medical center

ETHNICITY/CULTURE

- Mexican American

PREEXISTING CONDITIONS

COEXISTING CONDITIONS

- Strong familial predisposition; two brothers with colon cancer

LIFESTYLE

- Utility employee
- Worked with asbestos for 28 years

COMMUNICATION

- English as a second language

DISABILITY

SOCIOECONOMIC STATUS

- Middle

SPIRITUAL/RELIGIOUS

- Catholic

PHARMACOLOGIC

PSYCHOSOCIAL

- Anxiety
- Depression
- Fatigue

LEGAL

- Work-related factor may result in compensation

ETHICAL

- Possibility of early retirement

ALTERNATIVE THERAPY

- St. John's Wort

PRIORITIZATION

- Initial interview
- Questions about genitourinary history

DELEGATION

- RN
- Client education

MODERATE

THE DIGESTIVE AND URINARY SYSTEMS

Level of difficulty: Moderate

Overview: This case involves the use of the nursing process, systems assessment, and critical thinking skills to provide optimum care while monitoring fluid and electrolyte status. Focus will be on family history, knowledge of the disease process, and the importance of compliance with treatment regimens.

Client Profile

Mr. G is a 52-year-old married male who is 5′10″ and weighs 190 pounds. He is employed by a major utility gas company. Mr. G is scheduled for an office visit with his family health care provider due to results of prior laboratory and diagnostic tests.

Case Study

Mr. G reports frequency of urination with reduction in urinary stream, dysuria, nocturia, change in bowel habits (constipation and occasional diarrhea), and a feeling of incomplete bowel emptying. He is concerned about the symptoms because of his family history of colon cancer. He also reports having had a history of gastric ulcers for five years and a family history cancer in both of his brothers. When questioned about his dietary habits, Mr. G reports maintaining a diet low in fiber, and high in fat, protein, and refined carbohydrates. However, every year since he turned 40, he has undergone an annual physical exam with his primary health care provider that includes digital/rectal examination His most recent digital/rectal examination was "abnormal;" his stools have been negative guaiac annually. At age 50, he had a proctosigmoidoscopy because of unusual constipation. His vital signs are:

Blood pressure: 140/78

Pulse: 80

Respirations: 18

Temperature: 98.4° F

During a rectal assessment at the clinic, a colon mass is located and will be staged as needed after further examination. The health care provider does a complete history and physical examination, then the client is scheduled for the following diagnostic tests: colonoscopy, serum for prostatic-specific antigen, acid phosphatase, alkaline phosphatase, and a transurethral ultrasonography (TRUS). Mr. G returns to the medical center on different dates to have the tests done. The tests are done as scheduled, and the results are received and reviewed by an oncologist and the medical team. Mr. G's laboratory results are:

Prostatic-specific antigen (PSA): 3.8 ng/mL

Acid phosphatase: 0.53 I/L

Serum alkaline phosphatase: 128 U/L

The TRUS reveals small tumors in the prostate gland. The oncologist, surgeon, and health care provider explain the results to Mr. G and make a diagnosis of prostate cancer Stage IIC. Plans for treatment are explained to the client and the decision is made for treatment. Mr. G remains in the Same Day Care oncology unit of the hospital for further instructions but will be sent home today.

The following are prescribed:

- External-beam irradiation with 175 rads × one week. Start first dose today then discharge to home.
- Oxybutynin chloride (Ditropan) 5 mg PO two times per day
- Return to Same Day Care oncology unit × six more days

Questions

1. Discuss the risk factors and pathophysiology of prostate cancer.

2. Discuss clinical manifestations of prostate cancer.

3. Discuss cultural and ethnic considerations for the male reproductive system.

4. Discuss diagnostic studies used to aid the confirmation of prostate cancer.

5. What are the purposes of the prescribed treatment and medication?

6. What are common adverse reactions to the prescribed treatment and medication?

7. Discuss other therapies that may be prescribed to treat prostate cancer.

8. Discuss surgical procedures used for Stage llC prostate cancer.

9. Discuss postoperative complications of prostate surgeries.

10. Discuss client education for prostate cancer.

Ulcerative Colitis

GENDER

F

AGE

35

SETTING

■ Hospital

ETHNICITY/CULTURE

■ White American

PREEXISTING CONDITIONS

■ Stress

COEXISTING CONDITIONS

■ Recurrent respiratory infection
■ Emotional stress

LIFESTYLE

■ Phlebotomy supervisor for a large private, nonprofit medical organization

COMMUNICATION

DISABILITY

SOCIOECONOMIC STATUS

■ Middle

SPIRITUAL/RELIGIOUS

■ Episcopalian

PHARMACOLOGIC

■ Mesalamine (Asacol)
■ Sulfasalazine (Azulfidine)
■ Metronidazole (Flagyl)

PSYCHOSOCIAL

■ Anxiety

LEGAL

ETHICAL

■ Is the quality of life optimal for a 35-year-old client with ulcerative colitis disease?

ALTERNATE THERAPY

■ Flaxseed
■ Vitamin C
■ Aloe vera

PRIORITIZATION

■ Assess pain
■ Maintain fluid and electrolyte balance

DELEGATION

■ RN
■ Client education

MODERATE

THE DIGESTIVE AND URINARY SYSTEMS

Level of difficulty: Moderate

Overview: This case involves accurate assessment of fluid loss, monitoring for signs of dehydration, and critical assessment of the abdomen for characteristics of bowel sounds, distention, and tenderness. It also involves prioritization in a triage situation to prevent serious complications.

Client Profile

Ms. V is a 35-year-old, unmarried phlebotomy supervisor for a large medical team. Ms. V is 5′10″ and weighs 120 pounds. She has a two-year history of inflammatory bowel disease and has been hospitalized twice for exacerbations of intermittent diarrhea and colicky pain in the right lower quadrant. She appears anxious upon arrival at the emergency department (ED) and verbalizes frustration with the recurring problems. Ms. V also reports occasional periods of depression, which she relates to the disease.

Case Study

Ms. V's fiancé accompanies her to the ED. Her vital signs on admission are:

Blood pressure: 110/68

Pulse: 104 and regular

Respirations: 20

Temperature: 101.2° F

Ms. V experienced ten bloody bowel movements of moderate amounts accompanied by localized abdominal pain prior to arriving in the ED. An intravenous line with IV fluid of D_5LR at 150 cc/hr is initiated via a peripheral venous access. Ms. V is later seen by the ED health care provider and a gastroenterologist for initial assessment and data collection to help determine her diagnosis. Ms. V is placed on "nothing by mouth" (NPO) status, except ice chips. Plans to insert a nasogastric tube if she vomits are discussed with the health care provider and nurse. Serum labs prescribed prior to invasive diagnostic work-up include: hematocrit, hemoglobin, white blood cell count, erythrocyte sedimentation rate, serum sodium, serum potassium, serum chloride, albumin, stool for occult blood, ova, parasites, culture, and sensitivity. Results of the serum labs are:

White blood cell (WBC) count: 12,000/mm³

Erythrocyte sedimentation rate (ESR): 24 mm/hr

Hemoglobin (Hgb): 15.2 g/dL

Hematocrit (Hct): 30.5%

Potassium (K+): 2.6 mEq/L

Blood urea nitrogen (BUN): 18 mg/dL

Sodium (Na): 134 mEq/L

Chloride (Cl⁻): 98 mEq/L

Creatinine: 0.09 mg/dL

A double-contrast barium enema with air contrast and colonoscopy with biopsies are discussed with Ms. V and will be scheduled for the next day if the vomiting and diarrhea subsides. The vomiting and diarrhea subside and the double-contrast barium enema and biopsies are done, which provide the definitive diagnosis of ulcerative colitis (UC). The results are reviewed by the radiologist, followed by discussion with the multidisciplinary team and the client, and the plan of care is initiated.

The following are prescribed:
- Mesalamine (Asacol) 800 mg PO three times per day
- Sulfasalazine (Azulfidine) 250 mg PO four times per day
- Metronidazole (Flagyl) 7.5 mg/kg IV q6h

- Loperamide (Imodium) 4 mg PO followed by 2 mg after each formed stool
- Potassium chloride (K-chloride) 10 mEq/100 mL IV × four doses, repeat serum potassium after last dose

Questions

1. What are common nursing diagnoses for the client with UC?

2. What are the expected findings of the barium enema with air contrast and endoscopy?

3. What is the purpose of intestinal biopsies in diagnosing UC?

4. What type of psychotherapy would be most effective for Ms. V at this time?

5. Discuss a serious cardiac complication that may develop due to Ms. V's low serum potassium level.

6. What are the purposes for the prescribed orders?

7. What are the most common adverse reactions, drug-to-drug, drug-to-food/herbal interactions of the prescribed medications?

8. Identify complementary and alternative therapies for clients with UC.

9. Discuss specific nursing intervention activities for clients receiving intravenous potassium replacement for hypokalemia.

10. Discuss community-based nursing care for clients with risk for hypokalemia being discharged to home.

Acute Renal Failure

GENDER

F

AGE

60

SETTING

- Hospital

ETHNICITY/CULTURE

- Black American

PREEXISTING CONDITIONS

- Hypertension
- Diabetes mellitus type 2

COEXISTING CONDITIONS

- Diabetes
- Hypertension

LIFESTYLE

- Housewife

COMMUNICATION

- Spanish and English

DISABILITY

- Yes

SOCIOECONOMIC STATUS

- Low

SPIRITUAL/RELIGIOUS

- Catholic

PHARMACOLOGIC

- Dopamine HcL
- Lantus (Insuline glargine)
- Human regular insulin (Humulin R)
- Nifedipine (Procardia)
- Furosemide (Lasix)
- Calcium carbonate (Os-cal)
- Digoxin (Lanoxin)
- Sodium polystyrene sulfonate (Kayexelate)

PSYCHOSOCIAL

- Depression

LEGAL

ETHICAL

- Is there an ethical dilemma of randomizing clients with ARF to a certain dialysis modality?

ALTERNATIVE THERAPY

- Prayer

PRIORITIZATION

- Determine risk factors for ARF
- Assess fluid balance
- Monitor serum potassium levels

DELEGATION

- RN
- Client education

MODERATE

THE DIGESTIVE AND URINARY SYSTEMS

Level of difficulty: Moderate

Overview: This case involves critical assessment of the client. The nurse must question the client about decrease in urinary output; history of hypertension; use of prescribed medications/herbals taken independently; history of constipation or diarrhea, anorexia, nausea or vomiting, and unusual fatigue. The case involves prioritization in a triage situation with other clients experiencing acute onset of other diseases. The nurse must use critical thinking in triaging clients in order of highest priority to avoid or manage complications that could develop. The nurse must be knowledgeable about sites of drug metabolism and must constantly monitor for unintended effects of prescribed drugs.

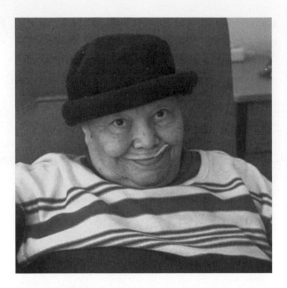

Client Profile

Ms. D is a 60-year-old client who lives in an apartment building in a "comfortable" two-bedroom apartment. Her significant others include her parents, who are alive and reside in a nursing home; and four younger brothers and one sister, all of whom are alive and well and have frequent contact with Ms. D. Her family history includes both parents having hypertension and a younger brother having type I diabetes for five years. Ms. D is 5′5″ and weighs 190 pounds.

Case Study

Ms. D is admitted to the hospital with complaints of increased fatigue, lethargy, and occasional confusion. After the initial interview, history, and physical examination by a registered nurse (RN) and a physician's assistant (PA), Ms. D is transferred from the triage area to a medical care unit. Vital signs in the emergency department (ED) are:

Blood pressure:160/98

Pulse: 78

Respirations: 16

Temperature: 98.5° F

Ms. D informs the receiving nurse in the medical unit that she is on lantus (Insulin glargine) ten units daily at bedtime, and does fingerstick glucose monitoring every four hours during the day. She admits being anxious because during the past two weeks she has experienced unusual dryness of the skin, which requires scratching. Ms. D decided to come to the hospital and goes to the ED because she believes she will get attention faster. When Ms. D is asked about the amount of urine voided since she awoke, she informs the receiving nurse and PA that since she has awakened, she has urinated a smaller amount within a seven-hour period when compared to other times. However, Ms. D believes the decrease in urinary output is related to her decrease in appetite, including fluids. Ms. D is currently taking furosemide 40 mg PO daily, captopril 50 mg PO two times per day for high blood pressure, and ibuprofen or naproxen occasionally for joint pains. She is also taking insulin for diabetes and ibuprofen PRN joint pain prescribed by her primary health care provider. Ms. D also reports a noted decrease in urinary output and unusual irritation frequently. She is admitted to the unit and placed on a cardiac monitor.

A peripheral intravenous line is inserted, and IV fluid of NaCL 0.45% at 75 mL/hr is initiated. The nurse continues with the physical assessment and auscultation of her heart sounds. There is S_3 gallop and bilateral rales over lung fields, especially at the bases, and +1 pedal edema at the ankles. Ms. D is placed in a semi-Fowler's position, and the nurse assigns a certified nursing assistant to remain with Ms. D, while she documents her findings. A chest X-ray is done and signs of congested heart failure are evident. Furosemide 40 mg IV is administered stat. Ms. D is seen by a health care provider and a history and physical examination are done, the history and assessment done by the nurse are reviewed, and the following diagnostic and laboratory tests are ordered: X-ray of the kidneys, ureters, and bladder (KUB); renal ultrasonography; and a cystoscopy. Ms. D's laboratory values are:

Blood urea nitrogen (BUN): 25 mg/dL

Creatinine: 2.8 mg/dL

Sodium (Na): 130 mEq/L

Potassium (K+): 6.8 mEq/L

Calcium: 8 mg/dL

Magnesium: 3 mEq/L

Phosphorous: 6 mg/dL

Glucose: 118 mg/dL

Urine specific gravity: 1.002

Urine sodium concentration: 48 mEq/L.

A consent is signed for a cystoscopy and central venous pressure catheter insertion. The catheter is inserted and an X-ray is negative for malposition of the catheter. Intravenous fluid is changed to Lactated Ringers at 75 mL/hr, and a foley catheter is inserted and attached to a urometer collecting bag. The results of the diagnostic and labs tests are received and reviewed by the health care provider: the KUB is negative for stones obstructing the renal pelvis, ureters or bladder; the renal ultrasonography is negative for urinary obstruction, but the renal calyces and collecting ducts are dilated, and tissue perfusion is impaired. The cystoscopy is negative for obstruction of the lower urinary tract. The medical doctor, the PA, the RN, an endocrinologist, and a cardiologist review the results of the diagnostic studies. A primary diagnosis of ARF is made, and secondary diagnosis of congested heart failure. The health care provider discusses the plan of care, including hemodialysis, with Ms. D. She is transferred to the medical intensive care unit (MICU), an electrocardiogram (EKG) is done, and the client is placed on continuous telemetry to monitor for life-threatening arrhythmias. Because of the current elevated serum potassium level, the EKG reveals tall, peaked T waves, widening of the QRS complex, and ST segment depression. Dopamine HcL (Intropin) infusion 2 microgram/kg is initiated.

The following are prescribed:
- Furosemide (Lasix) 40 mg IV q6h × 24 hours
- Nifedipine (Procardia) 20 mg PO three times per day
- Lantus (Insulin gargline) 10 units SC at bedtime
- Human regular insulin (Humulin R): Fingerstick sliding scale (FSS) q4h PRN for:

  Glucose less than 100 mg/dL, no insulin coverage; 100–140, two units SC; 141–180, four units SC; 181–220, six units SC; 221–260, eight units SC; 261–300, ten units SC; 301–340, twelve units SC; greater than 341, call the MD.

- Calcium carbonate (Os-cal) 4 g PO with meals
- Digoxin (Lanoxin) 125 mg PO every morning
- Sodium polystyrene sulfonate (Kayexalate) 15 g PO daily for potassium level greater than 5 mEq/L
- Monitor serum creatinine, BUN, serum sodium, potassium, glucose, hematocrit and hemoglobin, urine protein, and urine specific gravity daily.
- Dietary consultation, strict intake and output, record daily weight

Questions

1. Discuss your understanding of the medical diagnosis of ARF, considering all of the information provided in the case study, and the pathophysiology of ARF.

2. Discuss some of the common causes of ARF.

3. Discuss the phases that ARF progresses through.

4. What are the primary strategies of treatment for ARF?

5. What are common nursing diagnoses for ARF?

6. Briefly discuss the types and purpose of hemodialysis use to eliminate toxic factors from the blood to prevent fatal complications.

7. Including dopamine HcL, which was administered in the MICU, what are the purposes for the prescribed orders?

8. What are the most common adverse reactions to the prescribed medications?

9. Discuss the drug-to-drug and drug-to-food/herbal interactions for the prescribed medications.

10. Discuss the gerontologic considerations of ARF.

11. Discuss client education for ARF.

Appendicitis

GENDER

M

AGE

38

SETTING

- Hospital

ETHNICITY/CULTURE

- Black American/West Indian

PREEXISTING CONDITIONS

COEXISITING CONDITIONS

LIFESTYLE

- RN specializing in psychiatry

COMMUNICATION

DISABILITY

SOCIOECONOMIC STATUS

- Middle

SPIRITUAL/RELIGIOUS

- Anglican

PHARMACOLOGIC

- Ampicillin sodium/sulbactam sodium (Unasyn)
- Gentamicin sulfate (Garamycin)
- Metoclopramide HcL (Reglan)
- Metronidazole (Flagyl)
- Morphine sulfate (Duramorph)

PSYCHOSOCIAL

- Anxiety

LEGAL

ETHICAL

ALTERNATIVE THERAPY

PRIORITIZATION

- Assess and manage pain
- Prepare for surgery

DELEGATION

- RN

MODERATE

THE DIGESTIVE AND URINARY SYSTEMS

Level of difficulty: Moderate

Overview: This case involves critical thinking and focused assessment skills to prioritize care for a client with appendicitis with peritonitis. It involves accurate assessment of pain with specific identification of location of pain and thorough assessment and auscultation of the chest to rule out lower lobe pneumonia. The triage nurse should be skilled at detecting signs of septic shock that could occur with the client with ruptured appendix.

Client Profile

Mr. W is a 38-year-old registered nurse who has specialized in psychiatric nursing. He is 5′4″ and weighs 210 pounds. Mr. W is brought by a neighbor to the emergency department (ED), accompanied by his wife. The mode of transportation is a car.

Case Study

Mr. W denies past medical or surgical history. He reports that while preparing to leave for his place of employment, he had an unusually sharp pain in his abdomen. He tells the triage nurse that he had been having "on and off" pain in the abdominal area and that, at times, the pain was continuous. He said today he felt "unusually cool" but thought it was due to the weather. However, when the pain shifted to his right lower quadrant and remained localized at the area halfway between the umbilicus and the right iliac crest (McBurney's point), he informed his wife of the need to go the ED. On arrival at the ED, Mr. W is complaining of nausea, and begins vomiting. He is assisted to a stretcher, and immediately positions himself on his side with his right leg flexed. The ED health care provider is notified and the triage nurse continues to gather the history by focusing on Mr. W's description of the origin of the pain, intensity, and duration. Upon completion of the pain assessment, the nurse proceeds to perform a physical examination, using the system's approach, then examines the most tender quadrant of the abdomen last. The lungs are clear on auscultation and normal breath sounds are present, ruling out any relationship with the abdominal pain and lower lobe pneumonia. The ED nursing technician monitors the vital signs and reports:

Blood pressure: 110/70

Pulse: 80

Respirations: 18

Temperature: 100.0° F

The ED health care provider sees Mr. W and history and assessment examination are completed. Mr. W is transferred to a medical surgical unit in preparation for further evaluation and probable emergency surgery. He is given morphine sulfate 4 mg IM. He is on NPO ("nothing by mouth") status but has intravenous fluid 0.9% sodium chloride at 125 mL/hr. Electrocardiogram (EKG) and chest X-ray results are normal. Results from serum labs drawn on arrival to the ED reveal:

White blood cell (WBC) count: 20,000/mm³

Hematocrit (Hct): 30%

Hemoglobin (Hgb): 15 mg/dL

Urinalysis reveals hematuria, albuminuria, and pyuria. Blood culture reveals gram-negative anaerobic bacilli. Ultrasound study shows the presence of appendicitis. Diagnostic tests and lab results done in the ED are reviewed, and a diagnosis of appendicitis is confirmed. Mr. W is informed of the need for surgery, an order for type and cross match for two units of packed red blood cells (PRBCs) is placed, an informed consent is signed, and the operating room staff is notified. Ampicillin sodium/sulbactam sodium (Unasyn) 1 g IV is administered stat, and the client is waiting "on call" to the operating room for an appendectomy.

The following are prescribed:
- NPO, start IV fluid D %.45% NaCL at 125 mL per hour
- Metoclopramide HcL (Reglan) 10 mg IV q6h PRN. Dilute in 50 mL normal saline and infuse over 30 minutes.

- Morphine sulfate (Duramorph) 8 mg q4h PRN pain
- Ampicillin sodium/sulbactam sodium (Unasyn) 1.5 g IV × one before surgery
- Gentamicin sulfate (Garamycin) 80 mg loading dose IV × one before surgery
- Metronidazole (Flagyl) 15 mg/kg IV before surgery

Questions

1. Define appendicitis.

2. Discuss the etiology and pathophysiology of appendicitis.

3. Discuss the classic manifestations of appendicitis and some diseases that mimic appendicitis.

4. Discuss the complications associated with acute appendicitis.

5. Discuss the collaborative management for appendicitis.

6. What are common nursing diagnoses for appendicitis?

7. If the client starts to vomit, what interventions should be carried out by the nurse, in order of priority?

8. What are the purposes for the prescribed medications?

9. What are the most common adverse reactions to the prescribed medications?

10. Discuss the drug-to-drug and drug-to-food/herbal interactions for the prescribed medications.

CASE STUDY 7

Lower Gastrointestinal Bleeding

GENDER

M

AGE

70

SETTING

■ Hospital

ETHNICITY/CULTURE

■ Black American

PREEXISTING CONDITIONS

COEXISTING CONDITIONS

LIFESTYLE

■ Professional painter

COMMUNICATION

DISABILITY

SOCIOECONOMIC STATUS

■ Middle

SPIRITUAL/RELIGIOUS

■ Episcopalian

PHARMACOLOGIC

■ Aluminum hydroxide (Amphogel)
■ Misoprostol (Cytotec)
■ Ferrous sulfate (Feosol)

PSYCHOSOCIAL

■ Anxiety

LEGAL

ETHICAL

ALTERNATIVE THERAPY

PRIORITIZATION

■ Stop the bleeding
■ Increase tissue perfusion
■ Prevent shock

DELEGATION

■ RN
■ Client education

THE DIGESTIVE AND URINARY SYSTEMS

Level of difficulty: Moderate

Overview: This case involves a thorough account of the current problem, symptoms, and any treatments related to the current problem; exploration of characteristics associated with reported or overt symptoms and factors that may be the cause of symptoms; assessment for pain, a common problem with gastrointestinal (GI) tract disorders. Observation of the skin for discoloration, jaundice, or ecchymosis should be included in the assessment.

Client Profile

Mr. G is a 70-year-old male who travelled with his wife for a family reunion but upon arrival at the city of destination, he was taken from the airport to the emergency department (ED) of a city hospital because he had fainted in the parking lot of the airport after clearing customs. Mr. G is 5′9″ and weighs 204 pounds.

Case Study

Mr. G is brought from the airport by emergency medical services (EMS) to the ED, accompanied by his wife. On arrival, Mr. G is alert, and oriented to all stimuli. His vital signs are:

Blood pressure: 110/78

Pulse: 108

Respirations: 16

Temperature: 98.4° F

A nurse practitioner (NP) initiates the assessment. The sclera of both eyes are almost white, but his skin is dry and warm. His wife reports that he has not been eating as he usually does and he has slept much more than usual for the past three weeks. She also reports that his steps have been much slower than normal and he has not been as "jovial" as he usually is. Mr. G reports loss of appetite and a decrease in bowel movement, with only one bowel movement every other day (his usual is daily). He denies past medical or surgical history but informs the nurse that he has noticed that his bowel movement has been black and tarry, but he did not think anything about it. He reports taking "aspirin" for arthritic pain during the past six months. His heart sounds are normal, bilateral breath sounds are clear, and respirations are normal. His abdomen is soft and nontender to the touch, and bowel sounds are hyperactive. On rectal exam, there is dark-colored blood and tarry stool. Stool for guaiac is done and is positive for occult blood. There are no other abnormalities on rectal examination. Specimen is drawn and sent to the lab for hematocrit, hemoglobin, red blood cell count, partial thromboplastin time, activated partial thromboplastin time, serum iron, transferrin, and blood for type and cross match. A 12-lead electrocardiogram (EKG) is done and reveals normal sinus rhythm. A health care provider continues with the assessment after discussing the initial findings with the NP. An 18-gauge intravenous catheter is inserted and 0.9% NaCL is initiated at 100 mL per hour. A nasogastric tube (NGT) is inserted, and aspirate is analyzed for bleeding but is negative for the presence of blood. Results of the labs reveal:

Hematocrit (Hct): 24%

Hemoglobin (Hgb): 10 mg/dL

Red blood cell (RBC) count: 4.5/mm^3

Partial thromboplastin time (PTT): 48 seconds

Activated partial thromboplastin time (aPTT): 48 seconds

Serum iron: 50 mg/dL

Transferrin: 230 mg/dL

Mr. G is transferred to the surgical unit where he receives two units of packed red blood cells (PRBCs). Mr. G is prepared for a virtual colonoscopy by receiving two cleansing enemas before the procedure. After the transfusion, Mr. G. reports "feeling much better." The colonoscopy is done and reveals hemorrhoids and small gastric ulcers in the area of the lower GI tract. The multidisciplinary team discusses the findings of the diagnostic studies with Mr. G and plans to do a proctosigmoidoscopy at a later time, depending on his length of stay, since he is from "out of town." Post-transfusion labs reveal:

Hct: 26%

Hgb: 12 mg/dL

Post-transfusion vital signs are:

Blood pressure: 110/74

Pulse: 98

Respirations: 18

Temperature: 98.4°F

Because Mr. G is not from the state where he is hospitalized, he is discharged to home with referral to his primary health care provider for a proctosigmoidoscopy, further evaluation to rule out diverticular diseases and benign anorectal diseases, and to reevaluate hematologic and GI status. A diagnosis of lower GI bleeding is confirmed by clinical symptoms and the colonoscopy.

The following are prescribed on discharge:

- Aluminum hydroxide (Amphogel) 60 mL one to three hours after meals
- Ferrous sulfate (Feosol) 325 mg PO three times per day
- Misoprostol (Cytotec) 200 mcg/50 mg

Questions

1. Discuss common causes for lower GI bleeding in adults.

2. Discuss the purpose of the NGT inserted on admission, and nursing implications for persons with NGTs.

3. Discuss the potentially severe transfusion-related complications and the nursing implications.

4. What are common nursing diagnoses directly related to Mr. G's situation?

5. What are the purposes for the prescribed orders?

6. What are the most common adverse reactions, drug-to-drug, drug-to-food interactions of the prescribed medications?

7. Discuss other diagnostic tests the health care provider could have ordered to locate the source of bleeding.

8. Discuss the similarity and differences between invasive colonoscopy and virtual colonoscopy.

9. Discuss the nursing responsibilities for the client experiencing a proctosigmoidoscopy.

10. Discuss client education for lower GI bleeding.

Chronic Renal Failure (End-Stage Renal Disease)

GENDER

F

AGE

64

SETTING

■ Hospital

ETHNICITY/CULTURE

■ White American

PREEXISTING CONDITIONS

COEXISTING CONDITIONS

LIFESTYLE

■ Retired interior decorator

COMMUNICATION

DISABILITY

SOCIOECONOMIC STATUS

■ Middle

SPIRITUAL/RELIGIOUS

■ Presbyterian

PHARMACOLOGIC

■ Epoetin alfa recombinant (Epogen)
■ Calcium carbonate (Os-cal)
■ Aluminum hydroxide (Amphogel)
■ Nifedipine (Procardia)
■ Folic acid (Apo-Folic)
■ Ferrous sulfate (Feosol)
■ Ducosate sodium (Colace)
■ Furosemide (Lasix)

PSYCHOSOCIAL

■ Anxiety

LEGAL

ETHICAL

■ Do all clients with renal failure have an unconditional right to dialysis, given the cost of dialysis and the relative few who benefit from it?

ALTERNATIVE THERAPY

PRIORITIZATION

■ Complete history, including nutritional habits and current medications
■ Discuss urinary elimination in detail

DELEGATION

■ RN
■ CNA
■ Client education

THE DIGESTIVE AND URINARY SYSTEMS

Level of difficulty: Difficult

Overview: This case involves a thorough assessment of the client's condition, including current medications as well as careful systems assessment to prioritize care and prevent further complications and maintain kidney function and homeostasis for as long as possible. Accurate monitoring of blood pressure and serum potassium are critical since hypertension and hyperkalemia are common complications of end-stage renal disease (ESRD). Critical assessment of fluid status to identify imbalance is needed.

DIFFICULT

Client Profile

Mr. P, a 64-year-old retiree, is 4'10" and weighs 170 pounds. He shares a private home with his younger brother, who transported him to the emergency department (ED) of the hospital. On arrival, he complains of having had a headache for the past two hours. His vital signs are:

Blood pressure: 200/150

Pulse: 110

Respirations: 30

Temperature: 98.6° F

He is alert and oriented but is slow to respond to questions. He denies chest pain but reports nausea and feels he will vomit at anytime.

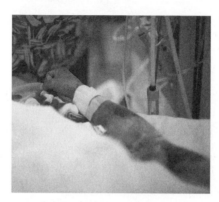

Double-lumen nasogastric tube

Case Study

Mr. P was diagnosed a year ago with end-stage renal failure secondary to hypertension, requiring treatment with hemodialysis. He is dialyzed at the clinic three times per week and is restricted to 1000 mL of fluid each day. He has a primary arteriovenous (AV) fistula in his left forearm (he is right handed). He reports current medications as:

Folic acid: 0.1 mg PO daily

Ferrous sulfate: 325 mg three times per day

Aluminum hydroxide: gel 500 mg PO twice

Erythropoietin alpha: self medicates with 50 units SC three times per week

Nifedipine: 30 mg PO three times per day

Mr. P reports not feeling his usual self, feeling tired on awakening this morning, and having difficulty getting out of bed. He is triaged and transferred to the medical intensive care (MICU), where an electrocardiogram (EKG) is done and shows sinus tachycardia and occasional unifocal premature ventricular contractions. Physical assessment reveals rales at the bases of the lungs and pitting edema of the lower extremities. Serum laboratory reports reveal:

Creatinine: 12 mg/dL

Blood urea nitrogen (BUN): 40 mg/dL

Sodium (Na): 150 mEq/L

Chloride: 100 mEq/L

Potassium (K+): 7.8 mEq/L

Phosphorous: 6.5 mg/dL

Calcium: 6 mg/dL

Hemoglobin (Hgb): 19 g/dL

Hematocrit (Hct): 28%

Glucose: 98 mg/dL

Arterial blood gas (ABG):

pH: 7.32

$PaCO_2$: 18 mm Hg

HCO_3: 8 mEq/L

PaO_2: 54

Mr. P is transferred to the dialysis unit soon after being transferred to the MICU and is dialyzed. A multidisciplinary team will participate in the overall plan of care, and the social worker, dietitian, and case manager will plan and coordinate home-care management.

The following are prescribed after the dialysis is completed:

- Folic acid (Apo-Folic) 0.1 mg PO daily
- Ferrous sulfate (Feosol) 325 mg PO three times per day
- Epoetin alfa (Epogen) 100 units/kg/dose SC three times per week
- Aluminum hydroxide gel (Amphogel) 500 mg PO four times per day
- Nifedipine (Procardia) 30mg PO three times per day
- Docusate sodium (Colace) 300 mg PO three times per day
- Calcium carbonate (Os-cal) 500 mg PO three times per day
- Furosemide (Lasix) 40 mg IV now and again in 4 hours

Questions

1. Discuss the pathophysiology of chronic renal failure, or ESRD.

2. Discuss the incidence, prevalence, and etiologies of ESRD in the United States.

3. Discuss why Mr. P was dialyzed soon after he was transferred to the MICU.

4. Discuss Mr. P's AV fistula and the purpose for it.

5. Discuss why the client is in metabolic acidosis.

6. What is the relationship between calcium, phosphorous, and chronic renal failure?

7. What are common nursing diagnoses for clients with ESRD?

8. Discuss hemodialysis (HD) versus peritoneal dialysis and why Mr. P was given hemodialysis instead of peritoneal dialysis.

9. What are the purposes for the prescribed medications?

10. What are the most common adverse reactions of the prescribed medications?

11. Discuss the drug-to-drug and drug-to-food/herbal interactions for the prescribed medications.

12. Discuss client education for ESRD.

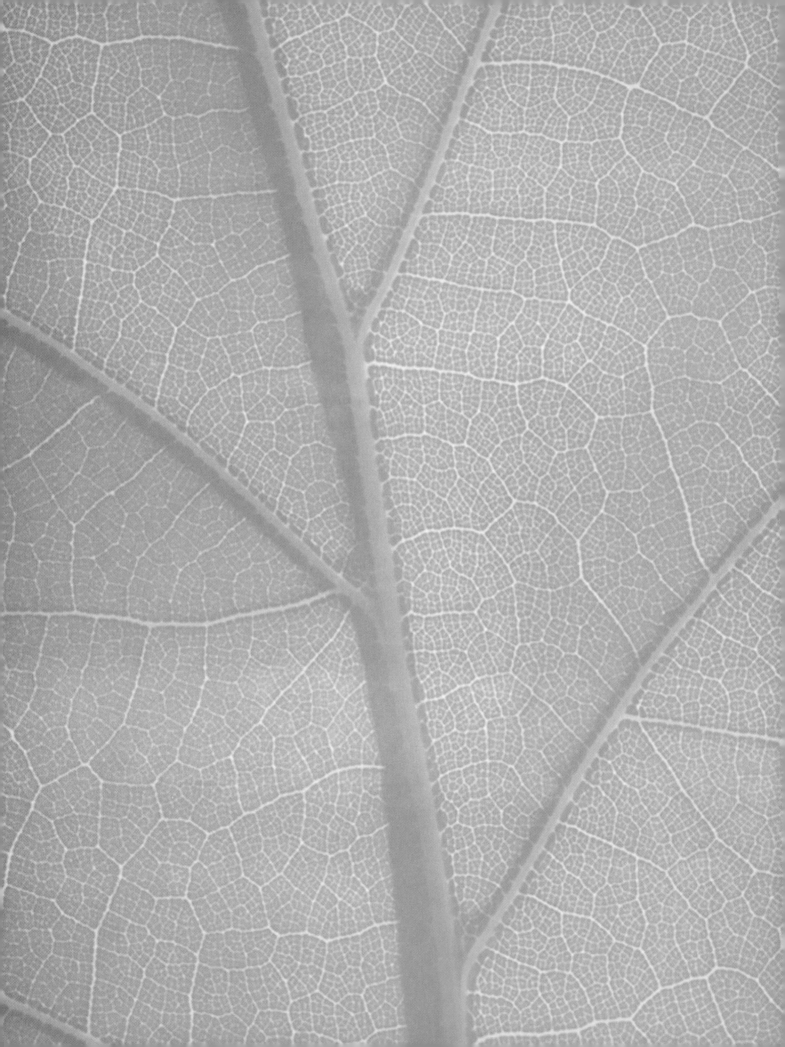

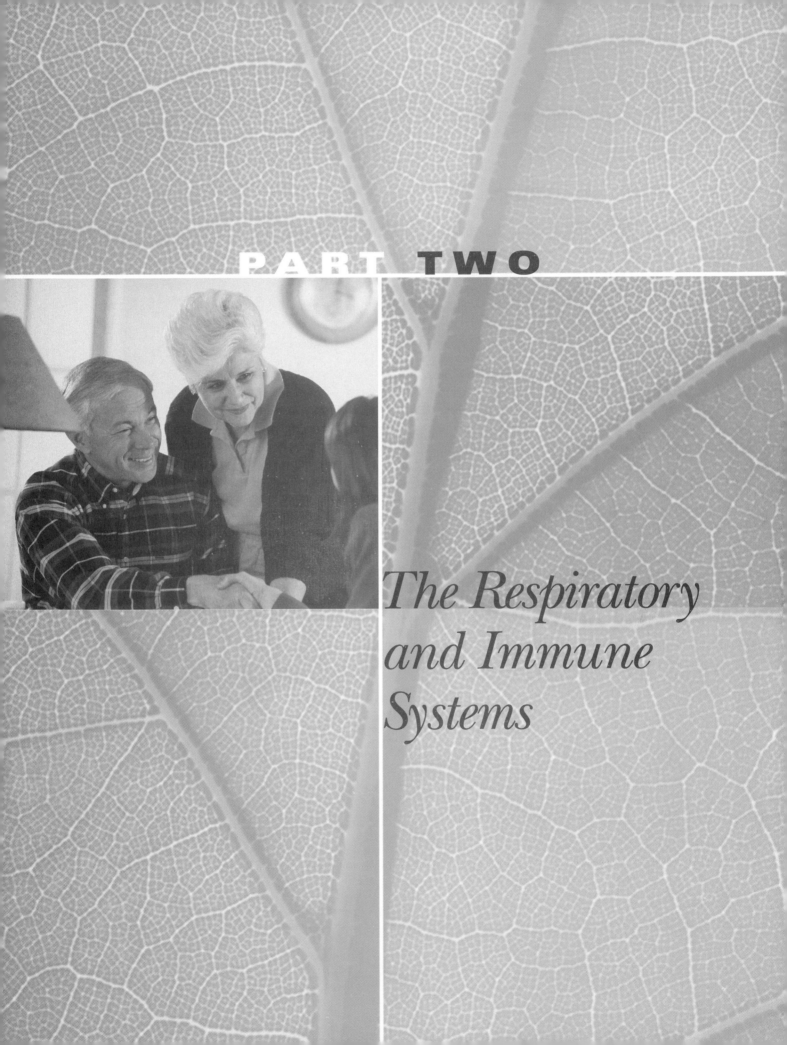

PART TWO

The Respiratory and Immune Systems

Chronic Bronchitis

GENDER

M

AGE

76

SETTING

- Skilled nursing facility

ETHNICITY/CULTURE

- White American

PREEXISTING CONDITIONS

COEXISTING CONDITIONS

- Viral infection
- Bacterial infection

LIFESTYLE

- Apartment building supervisor

COMMUNICATION

DISABILITY

- Decreased exercise tolerance

SOCIOECONOMIC STATUS

- Middle

SPIRITUAL/RELIGIOUS

- Protestant

PHARMACOLOGIC

- Albuterol (Proventil)
- Guaifenesin (Robitussin)
- Amoxicillin (Amoxil)
- Cefepime HcL (Maxipime)
- Ipratropium bromide (Atrovent)
- Acetaminophen (Tylenol)
- Oxygen

PSYCHOSOCIAL

- Anxiety
- Depression

LEGAL

ETHICAL

ALTERNATIVE THERAPY

PRIORITIZATION

- Maintain patent airway

DELEGATION

- RN
- Client education

THE RESPIRATORY AND IMMUNE SYSTEMS

Level of difficulty: Easy

Overview: This case involves prioritization of care to identify client's immediate needs and effective planning to have these needs met. The case also involves competence in identifying subtlety of grave changes with the client, such as absence of wheezing.

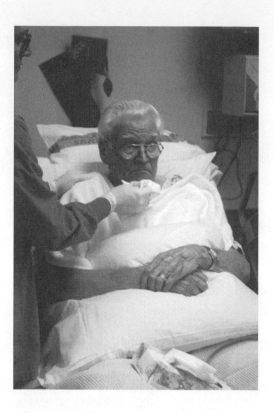

Client Profile

Mr. K, a 76-year-old male, is readmitted to the hospital's emergency department (ED) from a skilled nursing facility via an ambulette. On arrival, Mr. K shows signs of respiratory compromise as manifested by use of accessory muscles of the neck. The report from the nursing facility indicates that prior to this episode of respiratory impairment, Mr. K had been capable of carrying out basic activities of daily living such as combing his hair, mouth care, and dressing himself with only minimal assistance.

Case Study

During the past two weeks, Mr. K has been complaining of "stuffy" nose and has gradually begun to expectorate moderate amounts of respiratory secretions. The facility's health care provider is called because Mr. K has a temperature of 101°F and complains of chills even though the window of his room is closed and the air conditioning is off. His vital signs are:

Blood pressure: 124/86
Pulse: 80 and regular
Respirations: 20
Temperature: 101.0°F

Mr. K has a long history of cigarette smoking. On admission, he has thick, productive cough. The licensed practical nurse accompanying him informs the triage nurse that the cough has been unusually productive for more than one month, and Mr. K has had elevation of temperature of 101°F in the past that responded to Tylenol suppository. On auscultation, the ED nurse elicits loud rhonchi and wheezes. A complete history and physical is done, with physical findings that include clubbing of the fingers but no cyanosis or peripheral edema. A chest X-ray done on arrival to the ED reveals increased pulmonary congestion in the right lower lobe but no filtration or pleural effusion. Spirometry reveals airflow limitation with forced expiratory volume and forced vital capacity (FEV_1/FVC) 80%. Arterial blood gas (ABG) test reveals:

pH: 7.35
PO_2: 80
PCO_2: 47
HCO_3: 27

Mr. K is placed on two liters of oxygen via nasal cannula and is transferred to a respiratory unit of the hospital. On arrival at the unit, he continues to cough and, at times, coughs up blood-tinged sputum. A lab specimen is ordered, and results reveal sputum for culture and gram stain positive for Staphylococcus aureus and gram negative bacilli, white blood cell (WBC) with differential: WBC $14,000/mm^3$ and eosinophils $600/mm^3$. After the physical and laboratory data are reviewed, an admitting diagnosis of chronic bronchitis is confirmed.

The following are prescribed:

- Albuterol (Proventil) 2 puffs q4h and Ipratropium bromide (Atrovent) Soln, Inhl, 2.5 mL nebulization q4h
- Acetaminophen (Tylenol) 650 mg PO PRN temp greater than 100°
- Cefepime HcL (Maxipime) 1.5 g IV q12h
- Guaifenesin (Robitussin) 200 mg PRN q4h for cough
- D 5.45% NS IV infusion at 125 mL per hour

Questions

1. Discuss the cultural considerations for clients with chronic bronchitis related to history of cigarette smoking.

2. Discuss specific criteria used to diagnose chronic bronchitis.

3. Discuss the classic findings of clients with chronic bronchitis.

4. What are common nursing diagnoses for clients with chronic bronchitis?

5. What are the key features of cor pulmonale (right-sided heart failure), a complication of chronic bronchitis?

6. Discuss the breathing patterns commonly seen in clients with respiratory muscle fatigue.

7. What are the purposes for the prescribed orders?

8. What are the most common adverse reactions to the prescribed medications?

9. Discuss the drug-to-drug and drug-to-food/herbal interactions for the prescribed medications.

10. Discuss the key elements of stepped therapy for clients with chronic bronchitis.

11. What are the complementary and alternative therapies that help clients control dyspneic episodes?

CASE STUDY 2

Human Immunodeficiency Virus Infection (CDC Category A)

GENDER

F

AGE

32

SETTING

- Community clinic, a tertiary care center of a medical center

ETHNICITY/CULTURE

- Black South African

PREEXISTING CONDITIONS

COEXISTING CONDITIONS

LIFESTYLE

- Elementary school teacher

COMMUNICATION

- Xhosa and English as a second language

DISABILITY

SOCIOECONOMIC STATUS

- Middle

SPIRITUAL/RELIGIOUS

- Catholic

PHARMACOLOGIC

- Abacavir sulfate (Ziagen)
- Ritonavir (Norvir)
- Lamivudine/Zidovudine (Combivir)

PSYCHOSOCIAL

- Anxiety

LEGAL

- Client does not have the right not to release the names of those who may have contracted the disease from her.

ETHICAL

- Confidentiality—HIV is a reportable disease that carries a stigma.

ALTERNATIVE THERAPY

- Prayer
- Herbal medicines

PRIORITIZATION

- Maintain confidentiality
- Prepare for diagnostic tests

DELEGATION

- RN
- Client education

THE RESPIRATORY AND IMMUNE SYSTEMS

Level of difficulty: Easy

Overview: This case involves a thorough psychosocial and systems assessment and the use of optimum therapeutic communication to develop a sense of trust between client and health care providers. Room assignment is important due to the stigma of human immunodeficiency virus (HIV) and the client's lack of awareness of varying cultural views of the disease.

Client Profile

Ms. J is a 32-year-old female from Johannesburg, South Africa. She is vacationing with relatives who have resided in the United States for the past 40 years. Ms. J is accompanied by a cousin, a registered nurse, to the community center of a major city.

Case Study

On arrival at the clinic, Ms. J is restless as she waits for the next available nurse. During the initial interview, Ms. J informs the nurse that she is sexually active, practicing unprotected sex because she has been dating only her high-school sweetheart for years. Her reasons for seeking medical assistance are related to recent flu-like symptoms, including headache, fatigue, and occasional night sweats. Her report of unprotected sex and country of origin suggests the possibility of an early stage of human immunodeficiency virus (HIV). Her vital signs are:

Blood pressure: 150/98

Pulse: 120

Respirations: 22 and shallow

Temperature: 98.4° F

Ms. A is initially seen in the triage area of the ED by a nurse practitioner (NP), who notifies the ED physician of Ms. A's arrival and presenting symptoms. After the NP completes the history and physical, it is determined that Ms. J will need to return to the hospital for further evaluation. The NP, in collaboration with the clinic physician, assigns a tentative diagnosis of HIV to Ms. J, who is seen by a counselor and will return to the clinic in three weeks for a follow-up report on lab tests, then will see the primary health care provider at the hospital for a conclusive diagnosis. Lab results reveal CD4+/CD8 cell count 400 CD4+ cells/mm³ of blood. Enzyme linked immunosorbent assay (ELISA) and Western Blot tests are positive for HIV, chest X-ray reveals normal lung field, and structures within the thorax are normal. Purified protein derivative (PPD) injection is administered, is read in 72 hours, and is negative for tuberculosis. The health care provider and NP review the diagnostic reports and the laboratory data and confirm the diagnosis of HIV. The findings are discussed with the client, after which the health care provider and NP spend much time listening to the client and allowing verbalization of feelings about the diagnosis. Request for consultation with a psychiatrist and social worker is submitted. The HIPPA (Health Insurance Portability and Accountability Act of 1996) form is discussed with and signed by the client. A copy of the form is given to the client.

The following are prescribed:

- Abacavir sulfate (Ziagen) 300 mg PO two times per day
- Ritonavir (Norvir) 600 mg PO two times per day
- Lamivudine/zidovudine (Combivir) one combination tablet (150 mg lamivudine/300 mg zidovudine) PO two times per day
- Epzicom (Abacavir) 300 mg PO two times per day

Questions

1. Discuss the pathophysiology of HIV infection.

2. Discuss the modes of transmission that have remained constant throughout the course of the HIV pandemic.

3. Discuss the protozoal infections detected in persons with HIV.

4. Discuss how HIV is classified.

5. Discuss the clinical manifestations of HIV and how the infection is diagnosed.

6. List common nursing diagnoses for clients with HIV infection diseases.

7. Discuss highly active antiretroviral therapy (HAART) and whether the prescribed medications meet its criteria.

8. What are the purposes for the prescribed medications?

9. What are the most common adverse reactions of the prescribed medications?

10. Discuss the drug-to-drug and drug-to-food/herbal interactions for the prescribed medications.

11. Discuss the importance of the client seeing an HIV social worker before leaving the clinic.

12. Discuss dietary management for the person with HIV.

Pulmonary Tuberculosis

GENDER

M

AGE

50

SETTING

- Hospital

ETHNICITY/CULTURE

- White American

PREEXISTING CONDITIONS

COEXISTING CONDITIONS

LIFESTYLE

- Unemployed for five years
- Consumes beer or vodka daily

COMMUNICATION

DISABILITY

SOCIOECONOMIC STATUS

- Low

SPIRITUAL/RELIGIOUS

- Catholic

PHARMACOLOGIC

- Isoniazid (Nydrazid)
- Pyridoxine HcL (Aminoxin)
- Pyrazinamide (Tebrazid)
- Rifampin (Rifadin)
- Streptomycin sulfate (Streptomycin)
- Megestrol acetate (Megace)

PSYCHOSOCIAL

- Anxiety

LEGAL

- The client does not have the right to refuse providing names of persons who may have contracted the disease.

ETHICAL

- Cases of TB must be reported.
- Client's concern for confidentiality must still be addressed appropriately.

ALTERNATIVE THERAPY

PRIORITIZATION

- Private room
- Respiratory isolation
- Arrest TB process

DELEGATION

- RN
- Client education

THE RESPIRATORY AND IMMUNE SYSTEMS

Level of difficulty: Easy

Overview: This case involves a thorough assessment of the client's respiratory status, including social history and past exposure to tuberculosis (TB); the client's native country; and travel to foreign countries prior to migrating to the United States.

Client Profile

Mr. B is a 50-year-old male who is brought to the hospital emergency department (ED) by emergency medical service (EMS) from a community clinic after having bouts of vomiting while waiting to be seen by a health care provider.

Case Study

Mr. B's vital signs on arrival to the ED are:

> Blood pressure: 130/78
> Pulse: 78
> Respirations: 20
> Temperature: 99.0° F

He is known at the hospital; he frequently comes to the hospital's ED in a state of stupor or is taken by EMS because he has fallen while walking in the street. Today, he is coherent, responding to questions appropriately. Mr. B is 5'8" and weighs 110 pounds. Social history reveals he is a high school graduate who worked as a bookkeeper for a trucking company. He has been unemployed for the past five years. His social history reveals cigarette smoking for 40 years; he has smoked two packs per day for 20 years. He is an undiagnosed alcoholic, a former cocaine and marijuana user, and was "detoxed" from the cocaine six years ago. He denies having used marijuana during the past eight years. Mr. B also reports infrequent feelings of depression and noted weight loss for the past two months. He has never been married but has a son whom he has not seen for several years. Mr. B is currently taking Megestrol acetate 200 mg PO every six hours as prescribed by a health care provider at the clinic he attends and reports compliance with the medication. The health care provider in the ED continues with the history and physical examination and gathers from Mr. B that he has been experiencing a dry cough and occasional night sweats. Mr. B is transferred from the ED to the respiratory unit, with written orders to place him on respiratory isolation. On arrival at the unit, he is placed in a single room, and respiratory precaution signs are initiated on the outside of the door that leads to his room. The pulmonologist meets with Mr. B on the unit and, after further gathering of data, orders: sputum for acid fast bacilli (AFB) X three sputum culture, Mantoux test with 0.1 ml of PPD intradermally, and chest X-ray. The results for the diagnostic tests are positive for the mycobacterium bacillus, and the diagnosis of pulmonary tuberculosis is confirmed.

The following are prescribed:

- Isoniazid (Nydrazid) (INH) 300 mg PO daily
- Rifampin (Rifadin) (RMP) 600 mg PO daily
- Pyrazinamide (PZA) (Tebrazid) 30 mg/kg PO daily
- Streptomycin sulfate (Streptomycin) 15 mg/kg IM single dose
- Pyridoxine HcL (Aminoxin) 100 mg PO daily
- Megestrol acetate (Megace) 200 mg PO q6h

Questions

1. Discuss the incidence and prevalence of pulmonary TB.

2. Discuss the etiology and pathophysiology of TB.

3. What are the risk factors for TB?

4. Discuss the Centers for Disease Control (CDC) recommendations for preventing transmission of TB in health care settings.

5. Discuss the common clinical manifestations of clients with TB and how they reflect the pathophysiology of TB.

6. Discuss the gerontologic considerations for TB.

7. Discuss the specific diagnostic studies used to confirm TB.

8. What are the purposes for the prescribed medications?

9. What are the most common adverse reactions of the prescribed medications?

10. Discuss the drug-to-drug and drug-to-food/herbal interactions for the prescribed medications.

11. Discuss the potential complications for the client with TB.

12. Discuss client education for TB.

CASE STUDY 4

Pulmonary Empyema

GENDER

M

AGE

55

SETTING

- Hospital

ETHNICITY/CULTURE

- Black American

PREEXISTING CONDITIONS

- Pericarditis

COEXISTING CONDITIONS

- Renal failure

LIFESTYLE

- Retired

COMMUNICATION

DISABILITY

SOCIOECONOMIC STATUS

- Low

SPIRITUAL/RELIGIOUS

- Baptist

PHARMACOLOGIC

- Cefuroxime sodium (Zinacef)
- Gentamicin sulfate (Garamycin)
- Morphine sulfate (Duramorph)
- Rabeprazole sodium (Aciphex)

PSYCHOSOCIAL

LEGAL

- Are there federal or state supplemental resources to cover hospital expenses for self-employed retired persons?

ETHICAL

- Insufficient Social Security income should not be a deterrent for quality health care.

ALTERNATIVE THERAPY

- Prayer

PRIORITIZATION

- Antibiotic therapy

DELEGATION

- RN
- Client education

THE RESPIRATORY AND IMMUNE SYSTEMS

Level of difficulty: Easy

Overview: This case involves the use of collaborative management and history assessment to determine recent febrile illness, chest pain, dyspnea, or unusual cough. The nurse must be skilled in managing clients in need of thoracic procedures and competent in respiratory assessment and caring for clients with chest tubes to underwater seal drainage.

Client Profile

Mr. J, a 55-year-old male and retired self-employed carpenter, is readmitted to the hospital after being discharged two weeks ago. He is 5′10″ and weighs 230 pounds. At readmission he complains of pleuritic chest pain and generalized weakness. His vital signs on admission are:

Blood pressure: 150/90
Pulse: 100
Respirations: 30
Temperature: 101.0° F

Case Study

On physical assessment, Mr. J's chest wall motion is reduced, palpation and percussion reveal flat sounds, and breath sounds are decreased. Medical history reveals history of hypertension, past history of lung abscess and bacterial pneumonia, past history of pulmonary tuberculosis, recurrent left pneumothorax, and frequent upper respiratory infections. Mr. J reports gastric ulcer, which he relates to alcohol intake for several years, and allergies to contrast dye, radiographic dye, and thorazine. His social history involves several years of cigarette smoking. A chest X-ray is ordered and confirms pleural effusion. The health care provider determines the need to remove pleural fluid and explains the purpose and plan to Mr. J. An informed consent for a thoracentesis is signed by the client. The thoracentesis is done, and pleural fluid is sent to the lab for color, red blood cell count, white blood cell count and differential, and glucose and protein levels. The results are:

Appearance: cloudy
Red blood cell (RBC) count: $>1000/mm^3$
White blood cell (WBC) count: $>1000/mm^3$
pH: <7.4
Glucose: 68 mg/dL
Protein: >3.0 g/dL

A gram stain and acid fast stain are ordered and yields gram-negative species. Blood is positive for Staphylococcus aureus, and WBC is $15,000/mm^3$. A diagnosis of pulmonary empyema is confirmed and a treatment plan is discussed with Mr. J that includes the placement of chest tubes attached to water-seal drainage and wall suction.

The following are prescribed:

- Cefuroxime sodium (Zinacef) 1.5 g IV before the procedure/750 mg IV q8h × 24 hours
- Gentamicin sulfate (Garamycin) 2.5 mg/kg IV q8h
- Morphine sulfate (Duramorph) 2 mg IV q1–2h PRN
- Rabeprazole sodium (Aciphex) 60 mg PO once daily
- Chest tube to 20 cm wall suction via Pleur-evac

Questions

1. Discuss the pathophysiology of pulmonary empyema.

2. Discuss the findings on auscultation if pleural effusion is present with empyema.

3. What are management strategies for clients with pulmonary empyema?

4. Discuss pleural abnormalities as they relate to pulmonary empyema.

5. How would the health care provider determine that the client is experiencing compression of lung tissue due to the effusion?

6. What are the purposes for the prescribed medications?

7. What are the most common adverse reactions, drug-to-drug, drug-to-food/herbal interactions of the prescribed medications?

8. A tube thoracotomy is done, with chest tube for drainage. What are specific nursing interventions for managing chest drainage systems?

9. What are common nursing diagnoses for post–chest tube insertion?

10. Discuss client education for pulmonary empyema.

CASE STUDY 5

Non-Small Cell Adenocarcinoma of the Right Lung

GENDER

F

AGE

60

SETTING

- Hospital

ETHNICITY/CULTURE

- African/Nigerian

PREEXISTING CONDITIONS

- Recurrent pneumonias
- Pulmonary fibrosis

COEXISTING CONDITIONS

- Chronic obstructive pulmonary disease

LIFESTYLE

- Smoked three packs of cigarettes per day for 15 years

COMMUNICATION

DISABILITY

SOCIOECONOMIC STATUS

- Middle

SPIRITUAL/RELIGIOUS

- Attends Sunday Mass
- Spiritual counseling

PHARMACOLOGIC

- Ibuprofen (Motrin)
- Vinorelbine tartrate (Navelbine)
- Ondansetron HcL (Zofran)

PSYCHOSOCIAL

- Anxiety
- Fear
- Denial

LEGAL

ETHICAL

- Is it a nurse's responsibility to educate clients and others on the dangers of "secondhand smoke"?

ALTERNATIVE THERAPY

- Meditation
- Herbalism

PRIORITIZATION

- Reduce anxiety
- Prepare client for diagnostic tests

DELEGATION

- RN certified in oncology management
- Client education

THE RESPIRATORY AND IMMUNE SYSTEMS

Level of difficulty: Moderate

Overview: This case involves a thorough assessment of the client's condition, past medical history, social habits, and current medications including herbal and over-the-counter drugs. The nurse must use critical thinking and prioritization to meet the immediate needs of clients who are diagnosed with different types of cancer at different stages of progression. Nurses must be vigilant with assessment skills when caring for clients receiving chemotherapeutic agents that suppress bone marrow.

Client Profile

Ms. Y is a 60-year-old female who is admitted by her primary health care provider to the hospital after her annual physical examination. Ms. Y has never been married and has been unemployed for the past three years. She was employed as a "private" home health aide, but after the death of that client, she was unable to find employment.

Case Study

During the initial nurse interview, Ms. Y reports seeking her primary health care provider's advice because of a persistent cough for the past month. Ms. Y reports a history of smoking three packs of cigarettes per day for 15 years. Ms. Y admits to being anxious but does not believe she has cancer. She denies weight loss or unusual physical changes except the unusual cough. She reports occasional use of Advil (ibuprofen) for infrequent headaches and use of herbal medicines, especially at breakfast and before retiring to bed. Admission vital signs are:

> Blood pressure: 140/84
>
> Pulse: 80
>
> Respirations: 18
>
> Temperature: 98.2° F

Auscultation reveals unilateral wheeze in the right lower lobe of the lung. Respiratory assessment is occasionally interrupted because of her need to cough. After the physical assessment is complete, the following diagnostic studies and labs are prescribed: cytologic examination of sputum; chest X-ray; pulmonary function tests (PFTs); computed tomography (CT) scan of the lung; positron emission test (PET); serum sodium, potassium (K+), and calcium, platelet count, hematocrit, hemoglobin, white blood cell count, and creatinine. The results of the diagnostic tests reveal: sputum for cytology with malignant cells; chest X-ray shows lesion on the right lung; vital capacity (VC) is 75%, FEV_1 80%, FEF 68%; CT scan identifies the lesion and scans and measures it at 10 cm; PET is negative for metastasis. Results of the serum labs are:

> Sodium (Na): 133
>
> Potassium (K+): 4.2
>
> Calcium: 8.4
>
> Platelet count (PLT): 2,500,153
>
> Hematocrit (Hct): 32.8%
>
> Hemoglobin (Hgb): 11.5 g/dL
>
> White blood cell (WBC) count: 10,000/mm^3
>
> Creatinine: 0.9 mg/dL

After the diagnostic tests and lab results are reviewed and discussed with the medical, surgical, and oncology teams, a diagnosis of non–small squamous cell adenocarcinoma of the right lung is made. The findings are discussed and explained with Ms. Y, and a decision for plan of care is made. Serum sodium, calcium, complete blood count will be done twice weekly.

The following are prescribed:

- Vinorelbine tartrate (Navelbine) 30 mg/m² weekly at oncology clinic
- Ondansetron HcL (Zofran) 8 mg PO 30 minutes before chemotherapy

Questions

1. Discuss the pathophysiology of lung cancer.

2. Compare tobacco smoke, secondhand smoke, and environmental and occupational exposure and their effects on the development of lung cancer.

3. Discuss non-small cell lung cancer.

4. Discuss the clinical manifestations of lung cancer.

5. Discuss the different stages of lung cancer as designated by the tumor-mode-metastasis (TNM) classification system.

6. Discuss diagnostic tests use to confirm lung cancer.

7. What are the purposes for the prescribed orders?

8. What are the most common adverse reactions, drug-to-drug, drug-to-food/herbal interactions of the prescribed medications?

9. What process does the nurse use when administering medications to this client?

10. Discuss client education for lung cancer.

Pulmonary Emphysema

GENDER

M

AGE

62

SETTING

- Hospital

ETHNICITY/CULTURE

- Italian American

PREEXISTING CONDITIONS

- History of cigarette smoking

COEXISTING CONDITIONS

- Hyperinflated lung

LIFESTYLE

- Supervisor, 20 years in garment industry

COMMUNICATION

DISABILITY

- Easy fatigability
- Dyspnea on slight exertion

SOCIOECONOMIC STATUS

- Middle

SPIRITUAL/RELIGIOUS

- Catholic

PHARMACOLOGIC

- Theophylline ethylenediamine
- Methylprednisolone sodium succinate (Solu-Medrol)
- Cromolyn sodium (Intal)
- Albuterol (Proventil)
- Ampicillin sodium/sulbactam sodium (Unasyn)
- Pneumococcal 0.5 mL and influenza vaccine
- Metered-dose inhaler – Albuterol (Proventil)

PSYCHOSOCIAL

- Depression
- Anxiety

LEGAL

ETHICAL

ALTERNATIVE THERAPY

- Fish oil
- Garlic

PRIORITIZATION

- Airway management
- Prevent respiratory failure

DELEGATION

- RN
- CNA

MODERATE

THE RESPIRATORY AND IMMUNE SYSTEMS

Level of difficulty: Moderate

Overview: This case involves a thorough assessment of the client's condition including recent exposure to risk factors, pattern of symptom development, past medical history, current medications, and available social and family support. It involves prioritization of care. The nurse must be skilled at assessing respiratory status and competent in managing respiratory emergencies. The certified nursing assistant (CNA) can take height and weight, vital signs, and assist with hygiene care as needed.

Client Profile

Mr. X is a 62-year-old thin, underweight male who is accompanied by his wife to the respiratory unit after brief triage in the emergency department (ED). His wife is in the waiting room of the unit while the receiving nurse makes Mr. X comfortable before initiating the history and physical.

Case Study

Report from the triage nurse indicates that on arrival to the ED, Mr. X demonstrates signs of mild anxiety but his chief complaint is "increased difficulty breathing after climbing three flights of stairs today." He reports that his breathing has become progressively worse to the point where it interferes with activities of daily living (ADL). He concludes by saying that the breathing is worse today, which is the reason he came to the ED. His vital signs are:

Blood pressure: 140/78

Pulse: 88

Respirations: 24

Temperature: 99.8° F

On assessment, he has a barrel chest and uses his accessory muscles of respiration to assist with breathing. He frequently does pursed-lip breathing during the interview and coughs and expectorates moderate amount of yellowish sputum. He has auscultatory rales at the base of the lung fields. His social history includes smoking three packs of cigarettes per day for 40 years.

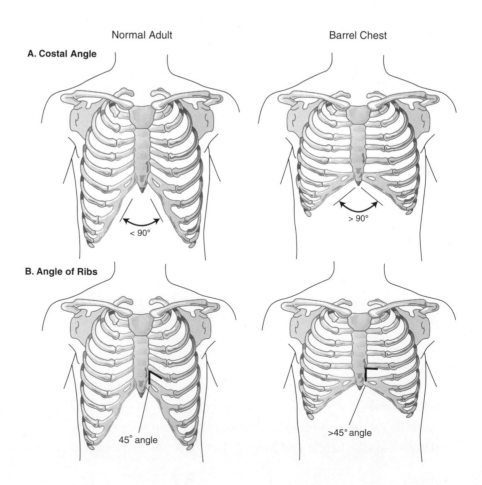

Normal Adult   Barrel Chest

A. Costal Angle

< 90°   > 90°

B. Angle of Ribs

45° angle   >45° angle

Mr. X reports not having gotten the pneumococcal and influenza vaccines for a long period of time but is not specific about the length of time. A health care provider completes the history and physical and orders a stat arterial blood gas (ABG) and complete blood count (CBC). The results of the ABG tests are:

pH: 7.36

$PaCO_2$: 48 mm Hg

PaO_2: 80%

HCO_3: 25

Complete blood count (CBC):

White blood cell (WBC) count: 7.1

Hematocrit (Hct): 38%

Hemoglobin (Hgb): 15 mg/dl

Two liters of oxygen via nasal cannula are initiated. A chest X-ray shows a flattened diaphragm but no infiltrates. Pulmonary function studies reveal FEV-1/FVC 60% and increased residual volume (RV). Sputum analysis identifies Haemophilus influenza. A diagnosis of chronic obstructive pulmonary disease (pulmonary emphysema) is confirmed. Mr. X is admitted to the hospital for respiratory and oxygen therapy and pharmacological therapy.

The following are prescribed:

- Albuterol (Proventil) aerosol metered-dose inhalant (MDI) two puffs stat and q4h PRN
- Oxygen/nasal cannula to maintain oxygen saturation greater than 89% but not to exceed two liters
- Dextrose 5% and 0.45% sodium chloride intravenous infusion at 100 ml/hr
- Theophylline ethylenediamine (with 20 mg theophylline, 25 mg aminophylline) 0.3 mg/kg/hr continuous intravenously administration
- Ampicillin sodium/sulbactam sodium (Unasyn) 1.5 gm IV q6h
- Cromolyn sodium (Intal) two metered sprays q6h
- Pneumococcal 0.5 mL single dose and influenza vaccine 0.5 mL single dose prior to discharge

Questions

1. Discuss the types of emphysema and the most common risk factor for the development of pulmonary emphysema.

2. Discuss the complications associated with emphysema.

3. Discuss the enzyme inhibitor that predisposes young clients who do not smoke to rapid development of lobular emphysema.

4. Pulmonary function tests (PFTs) are used to confirm pulmonary emphysema. What are the specific findings of the PFTs?

5. Discuss the clinical manifestations of pulmonary emphysema.

6. What are common nursing diagnoses for clients with pulmonary emphysema?

7. What are the purposes for the prescribed medications?

8. What are the most common adverse reactions of the prescribed medications?

9. Discuss the drug-to-drug and drug-to-food/herbal interactions of the prescribed medications.

10. Discuss the surgical approaches that might be used for the client with emphysema.

11. Discuss client education for pulmonary emphysema.

CASE STUDY 7

Acute Respiratory Distress Syndrome

GENDER

M

AGE

42

SETTING

- Hospital

ETHNICITY/CULTURE

- Black American

PREEXISTING CONDITIONS

COEXISTING CONDITIONS

LIFESTYLE

- Fireman

COMMUNICATION

DISABILITY

SOCIOECONOMIC STATUS

- Middle

SPIRITUAL/RELIGIOUS

- Catholic

PHARMACOLOGIC

- Lactated Ringers
- Enoxaparin (Lovenox)
- Midazolam HcL (Versed)
- Pancuronium
- bromide (Pavulon)
- Bumetanide (Bumex)

PSYCHOSOCIAL

- Anxiety

LEGAL

- Long-term financial support

ETHICAL

ALTERNATIVE THERAPY

PRIORITIZATION

- Maintain airway patency
- Maintain oxygenation

DELEGATION

- RN
- Client education

THE RESPIRATORY AND IMMUNE SYSTEMS

Level of difficulty: Difficult

Overview: This case involves a quick assessment of the client and presenting symptoms while maintaining airway patency. It involves prioritization of care to other clients when the burn client arrives on the unit. It involves a complete physical examination that includes the client's general appearance on arrival to the unit.

DIFFICULT

Client Profile

Mr. T is a 42-year-old firefighter assigned to an engine company located in a poor urban neighborhood. Mr. T has been acknowledged by the mayor of the city on three occasions for bravery, which includes going beyond the call of duty to save lives from actively burning buildings. One month ago, Mr. T was brought to the hospital emergency department (ED) for smoke inhalation after combating a fire for several hours. Mr. T was discharged and returned to work after clearance from his primary health care provider.

Case Study

Today, Mr. T is brought to the ED from his place of employment. On arrival at the ED, he is restless, complains of fatigue, headache, and difficulty breathing even when in an upright position. An arterial blood gas (ABG) test reveals:

pH: 7.30

PCO_2: 48

HCO_3^- done with a PaO_2 of 58

The test indicates respiratory acidosis. He is started on a non-rebreather mask and pulse oximeter to monitor oxygen saturation. Physical assessment by the nurse finds the use of accessory muscles with decreased breath sounds. Vital signs are:

Blood pressure: 100/72

Pulse: 114

Respirations: 22

Temperature: 99.4° F

Mr. T is 5'6" and weighs 205 pounds. Pulmonary function tests (PFTs) show decreased lung compliance with reduced vital capacity, minute volume and functional vital capacity. On auscultation of the lungs, the health care provider auscultates bilateral rales. Results of a chest X-ray done in the ED show diffuse haziness, "whited-out" (ground-glass) appearance of the lung. A repeat ABG reveals PaO_2 of 58 even after the implementation of four liters of oxygen. The client is intubated and placed on mechanical ventilation with positive-end expiratory pressure (PEEP) setting and placed in semi-Fowler's position. A pulmonary artery catheter is inserted. After review of physical findings, response to increase in oxygen, chest X-ray findings, and pulmonary capillary wedge pressure readings, the diagnosis of acute respiratory distress syndrome (ARDS) is made. Plans to initiate enteral feeding or parenteral nutrition (hyperalimentation) will be included in the treatment regimen.

The following are prescribed:

- Lactated Ringers 1,000 mLs at 125 mLs per hour
- Enoxaparin (Lovenox) injection 40 mg/0.4 ML SC daily
- Midazolam HcL (Versed) 0.02 mg/kg/h by continuous infusion
- Pancuronium bromide (Pavulon) 0.1 mg/kg IV initial dose
- Bumetanide (Bumex) 1 mg IV q6h for 24 hours

Questions

1. Discuss your understanding of the client's situation.

2. Discuss the pathophysiology of ARDS and the leading cause of death in clients with ARDS.

3. Discuss the usual cause of refractory hypoxemia in ARDS.

4. Discuss the purpose and benefits for the positive-end expiratory pressure (PEEP) setting on the ventilator.

5. Discuss the significance of pulmonary capillary wedge pressure (PCWP) in diagnosing ARDS.

6. What are common nursing diagnoses for clients with ARDS?

7. What are the purposes for the prescribed orders?

8. What are the most common adverse reactions of the prescribed medications?

9. Discuss the drug-to-drug and drug-to-food/herbal interactions of the prescribed medications.

10. Discuss essential nursing responsibilities when caring for mechanically ventilated clients on neuromuscular blockers.

Acquired Immunodeficiency Syndrome

GENDER

M

AGE

40

SETTING

- Hospital

ETHNICITY/CULTURE

- Hispanic American

PREEXISTING CONDITIONS

- HIV

COEXISTING CONDITIONS

- Peripheral neuropathy
- Hepatitis C
- Recurrent bacterial pneumonia

LIFESTYLE

- Cab driver for eight years

COMMUNICATION

- Spanish and English as a second language

DISABILITY

SOCIOECONOMIC STATUS

- Low

SPIRITUAL/RELIGIOUS

- Nondenominational

PHARMACOLOGIC

- Interferon alfa-2b (Intron A)
- Amikacin sulfate (Amikin)
- Bleomycin sulfate (Blenoxane)
- Nystatin (Mycostatin)
- Trimethoprim/sulfamethoxazole (Bactrim)

PSYCHOSOCIAL

- Fear

LEGAL

- Financial support
- Advance directives
- Counseling

ETHICAL

- Discrimination and denial have decreased national response to the AIDS epidemic. Strong, positive leadership for care and prevention is needed.

ALTERNATIVE THERAPY

- Aloe vera
- Echinacea

PRIORITIZATION

- Body substance isolation
- Confidentiality

DELEGATION

- RN
- LPN
- CNA

THE RESPIRATORY AND IMMUNE SYSTEMS

Level of difficulty: Difficult

Overview: This case involves thorough knowledge of the complexities of acquired immunodeficiency syndrome (AIDS) and is void of values that cloud professional approach to delegation of assignments and optimum care (i.e., immediate and general). The nurse must be familiar with the mix of medications usually prescribed for Persons With AIDS (PWAs). The licensed practical nurse (LPN) can administer medications as prescribed after the registered nurse (RN) has completed the initial assessment. The certified nursing assistant (CNA) can provide routine hygiene care and take vital signs, reporting abnormal readings to the LPN.

DIFFICULT

Client Profile

Mr. C is a 40-year-old male who was diagnosed with human immunodeficiency virus (HIV) five years ago and has been under outpatient medical supervision at a community health center affiliated with a medical center in the community in which he resides. Mr. C lives with his aunt, who is 68 years old and is his primary caregiver. Mr. C was seen in the outpatient clinic two weeks ago with complaints of nausea, vomiting, and diarrhea. Review of laboratory data and diagnostic studies from previous clinic visits indicate progression of the disease as evidenced by axilary adenopathy, decrease in CD+W cells of 300 mm^3, and oral candidiasis.

Case Study

Today Mr. C is seen in the outpatient clinic with complaints of severe diarrhea for two days, fever, and dry, productive cough. He reports being able to walk for approximately four feet without assistance but becomes extremely fatigued afterward. The nurse practitioner completes a history and physical examination and, after reviewing Mr. C's previous clinic records, refers him to the hospital for further evaluation and possible admission. At the hospital, Mr. C's vital signs are:

Blood pressure: 110/86

Pulse: 106

Respirations: 28 and shallow

Temperature: 102.6°F

He is sent from the admission's department to the AIDS unit and is assigned to a private room. Mr. C is placed on three liters of oxygen as per the unit's protocol. An arterial blood gas (ABG) is done and reveals:

pH: 7.35

pCO$_2$: 45

HCO$_3$: 28

pO$_2$: 78

The health care provider is notified, and the nurse initiates a brief history and physical, taking into consideration the physical and emotional state of the client. The nurse briefly discusses the Patient's Bill of Rights and the American Health Insurance Portability and Accountability Act of 1996 (HIPPA) with Mr. C and informs him that the documents will be given to him before the completion of the nurse's work schedule. Mr. C is seen by a health care provider who continues with the history and physical assessment then reviews Mr. C's medical records sent from the clinic, which include a diagnosis of AIDS. Current laboratory data from the clinic indicate values of: CD+4/CD8+ ratio less than 2 and CD4+ count of 200/mm^3, positive ELISA and Western Blot tests. Current blood cultures reveal Escherichia coli, Pseudomonas aeruginosa, and Klebsiella pneumoniae. After the multidisciplinary team reviews current data and physical assessment findings, an admitted with diagnosis is made for AIDS complicated with pneumocystis carinii pneumonia (PCP), cytomegalovirus (CMV) retinitis, Kaposi's sarcoma (KS), and oral candidiasis.

The following are prescribed:

- Interferon alfa-2b (Intron A) 20,000,000 IU/M^2 SC for five consecutive days pr week for four weeks
- Amikacin sulfate (Amikin) 7.5 mg/kg IV q12h

- Trimethoprim/sulfamethoxazole (Bactrim) 5mg/kg IV q6h for seven days and then PO q6h for seven days
- Bleomycin sulfate (Blenoxane) 0.5 U/kg IV × two weekly
- Nystatin suspension (Mycostatin) 500,000 U PO three times per day, swish and swallow
- Ondansetron 32 mg IV 30 minutes before bleomycin therapy
- Dextrose 5% in 0.45% normal saline at 125 mL/hr

Questions

1. Define PCP.

2. Discuss the clinical manifestations of PCP associated with AIDS.

3. Discuss the enteric pathogen that may occur in the stool of the client with AIDS.

4. Discuss the two cytokines that play an important role in AIDS-related wasting syndrome.

5. The Centers for Disease Control and Prevention (CDC) has included Kaposi's sarcoma (KS) in the classification of AIDS-related malignancies. Discuss how KS diagnosis is confirmed.

6. Discuss priority nursing diagnoses associated with AIDS.

7. What are the purposes for the prescribed medications?

8. What are the most common adverse reactions of the prescribed medications?

9. Discuss the drug-to-drug and drug-to-food/herbal interactions of the prescribed medications.

10. Discuss how the nurse can promote home- and community-based care.

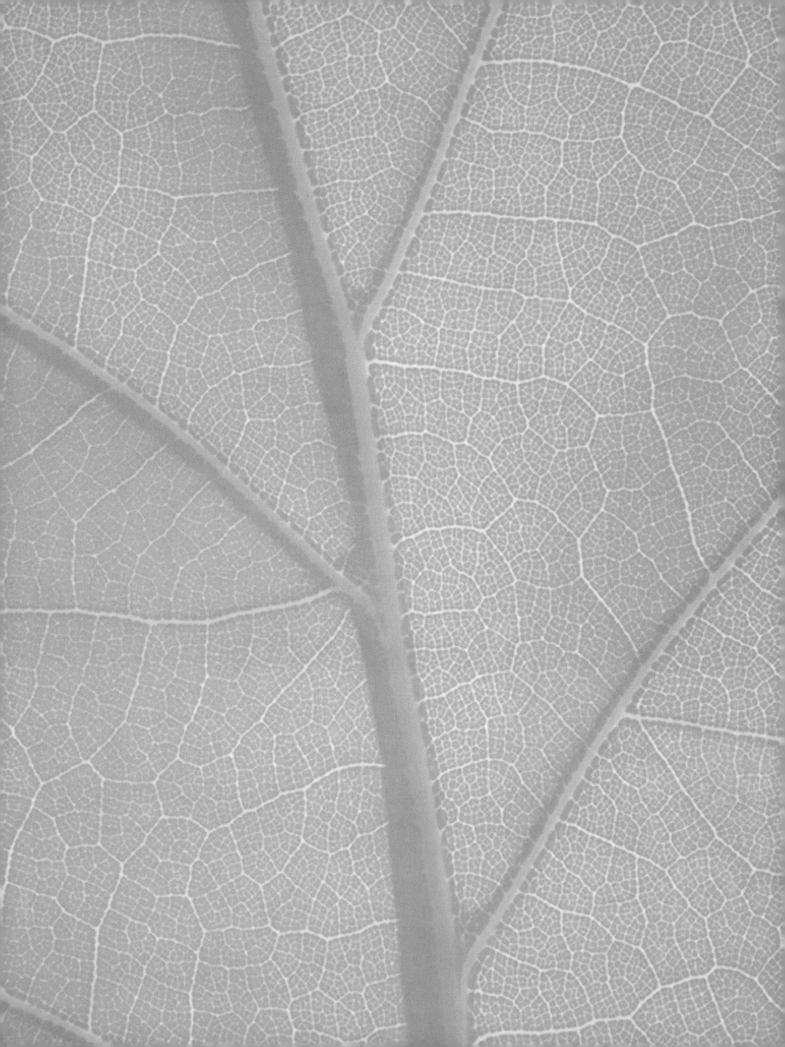

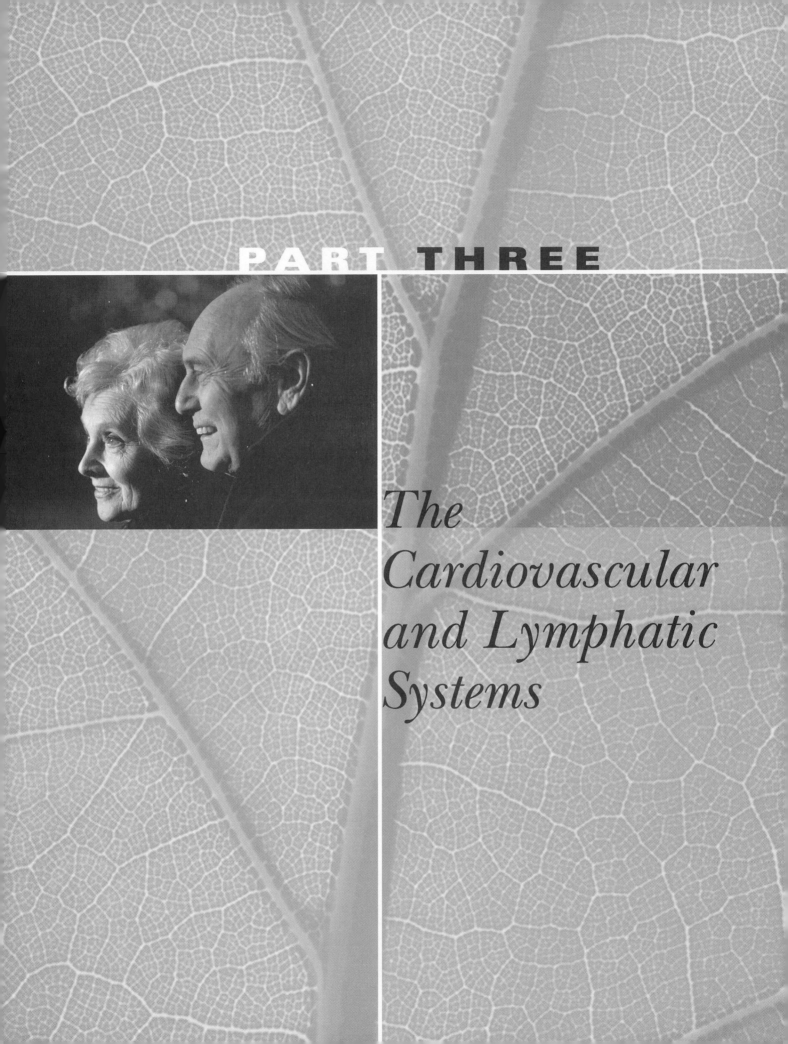

PART THREE

The Cardiovascular and Lymphatic Systems

CASE STUDY 1

Primary (Essential) Hypertension

GENDER

M

AGE

65

SETTING

- Hospital emergency department

ETHNICITY/CULTURE

- Black American

PREEXISTING CONDITIONS

- High blood pressure

COEXISTING CONDITIONS

- Family history: mother with history of hypertension died at age 70.

LIFESTYLE

- Part-time school bus driver. Work hours are 11:00–3:00, three days per week.
- Diet includes moderate amount of sodium.

COMMUNICATION

DISABILITY

SOCIOECONOMIC STATUS

- Low

SPIRITUAL/RELIGIOUS

- Baptist

PHARMACOLOGIC

- Furosemide (Lasix)
- Captopril (Capoten)
- Hydrochlorothiazide (HydroDIURIL)
- Spironolactone (Aldactone)
- Ezetimibe (Zetia)

PSYCHOSOCIAL

- Anxiety

LEGAL

ETHICAL

ALTERNATIVE THERAPY

- Listens to different kinds of music

PRIORITIZATION

- Interview
- Physical examination
- Evaluation of information
- Accurate monitoring of blood pressure

DELEGATION

- RN
- Client education

THE CARDIOVASCULAR AND LYMPHATIC SYSTEMS

Level of difficulty: Easy

Overview: This case involves understanding essential hypertension, monitoring blood pressure, administering prescribed medications, and clarifying the client's understanding of the disease. The case also involves client education and discharge planning with emphasis on follow-up care at the clinic or primary health care provider.

Client Profile

Mr. J is a 65-year-old male who has been visiting his primary health care provider yearly for annual examinations specifically related to history of mild congested heart failure (CHF). Over the past year, Mr. J notices that he gets infrequent headaches even though he is not stressed. Mr. J is 5′5″ and weighs 240 pounds.

Case Study

Mr. J reports a family history of hypertension and was diagnosed with primary hypertension at the age of 64. He reveals he likes foods that are high in sodium content. His father is alive and well, but his mother died at age 70 from a cerebral vascular accident related to hypertension. His social history reveals alcohol consumption of beer during the day and a glass of wine at dinner. Mr. J is seen by a nurse practitioner (NP) at the community clinic for complaints of headache and dizziness, which he reports experiencing while shopping at a department store. Upon admission, his vital signs are:

> Blood pressure: 190/110
>
> Pulse: 104 and regular
>
> Respirations: 18
>
> Temperature: 98.4° F

He is transferred to the local hospital's emergency department (ED) for further evaluation. On arrival at the ED, he is seen by an NP who initiates a systems assessment and finds his blood pressure reading to be 180/110 × two readings with the use of appropriate blood pressure cuff size. Mr. J reports current medications of captopril and metoprolol tartrate. He is kept in the ED for three hours on continuous telemetry while awaiting a bed on a medical unit. He is later transferred to a medical unit for further evaluations. Lab values are prescribed and include: urine for urinalysis, complete blood count, serum potassium (K+), sodium (Na), glucose, blood urea nitrogen (BUN), creatinine, cholesterol and triglyceride levels, serum aldosterone, and 24-hour urine aldosterone. His body mass index (BMI) is done and is 35, indicating that Mr. J is moderately obese for his height. The following are Mr. J's laboratory results:

> Urinalysis: negative
>
> White blood cell (WBC) count: 8,500 cells/mm^3
>
> Hematocrit (Hct): 33%
>
> Hemoglobin (Hgb): 15 g/dL
>
> Platelet count: 150,000 cells/mm^3
>
> Glucose: 80 mg/dL
>
> Blood urea nitrogen (BUN): 14 mg/dL
>
> Creatinine: 1.2 mg/dL
>
> Potassium (K+): 3.7 mEq/L
>
> Sodium (Na): 158 mEq/L
>
> Albumin: 3.4 gm/dL
>
> Calcium: 9 mg/dL
>
> Cholesterol: 218 mg/dL
>
> Triglyceride: 180 mg/dL
>
> Urine aldosterone: 30 ug/24 hr
>
> Serum aldosterone: 28 ng/dL

A fundoscopic examination of the eyes is done and indicates the retinal structures of the eyes are within normal limits. A 12-lead electrocardiogram (EKG) shows sinus rhythm, and a chest X-ray reveals normal heart size and normal lung structures. The dietitian sees the client and performs a three-day dietary recall, and plans to suggest a two-gram sodium diet to the multidisciplinary team. After the health care provider, pharmacist, NP, RN, and dietitian review the diagnostic tests and the laboratory data, a diagnosis of primary hypertension is confirmed.

The following are prescribed:

- Furosemide (Lasix) 40 mg IV stat
- Captopril (Capoten) 25 mg PO three times per day
- Hydrochlorothiazide (HydroDIURIL) 12.5 mg PO daily
- Spironolactone (Aldactone) 50 mg PO two times per day
- Ezetimibe (Zetia) 10 mg PO daily
- Two-gram sodium diet

Questions

1. What are specific cultural considerations in the United States for hypertension?

2. What are some common nursing diagnoses for clients with hypertension?

3. After the diagnosis of essential hypertension is confirmed with initial studies, what further evaluations are necessary?

4. What is the purpose of the registered dietitian in the multidisciplinary team conference with the client who is diagnosed with essential hypertension?

5. What are the purposes for the prescribed medications?

6. What are the most common adverse reactions of the prescribed medications?

7. Discuss drug-to-drug and drug-to-herbal interactions of the prescribed medications.

8. What is the ultimate goal of antihypertensive therapy?

9. Discuss the effects of angiotensin converting enzyme (ACE) on hypertension and nursing priority of care when caring for clients taking ACE inhibitor agents.

10. What are some complementary modalities clients with hypertension may use to decrease blood pressure?

11. Discuss client education for a captopril (Capoten) prescription upon discharge to home.

CASE STUDY 2

Coronary Artery Disease (Atherosclerosis)

GENDER

F

AGE

68

SETTING

■ Hospital's outpatient clinic

ETHNICITY/CULTURE

■ White American

PREEXISTING CONDITIONS

■ Obesity

COEXISTING CONDITIONS

■ Peripheral vascular disease

LIFESTYLE

■ Unemployed

COMMUNICATION

DISABILITY

SOCIOECONOMIC STATUS

■ Low

SPIRITUAL/RELIGIOUS

■ Anglican

PHARMACOLOGIC

■ Lipid-lowering agents
■ Diuretics
■ Cardiotonic
■ Vasodilator
■ Calcium-channel blocker
■ Anticoagulant

PSYCHOSOCIAL

■ Anxiety

LEGAL

■ Financial resources

ETHICAL

ALTERNATIVE THERAPY

PRIORITIZATION

■ Accurate systems assessment
■ Continuous telemetry

DELEGATION

■ RN
■ LPN
■ Client education

THE CARDIOVASCULAR AND LYMPHATIC SYSTEMS

Level of difficulty: Easy

Overview: The nurse will elicit appropriate nursing history to more accurately identify appropriate nursing diagnoses. The nurse also will use critical-thinking skills in identifying the client's immediate needs during triage. Client education is important before discharge from the hospital.

Client Profile

Ms. Z is a 68-year-old female who is 5′5″ and weighs 248 pounds. Her cardiologist refers her to the clinic of the community hospital after several complaints of fatigue and decrease in energy over the past month.

Case Study

Ms. Z is seen in the hospital outpatient clinic following the cardiologist's referral. She denies chest pain or palpitations on admission but reports frequent episodes of dizziness and inability to concentrate for "long periods of time." Her past medical history (PMH) includes hypercholesterolemia, chronic atrial fibrillation, episodes of syncope, occasional anginal type pain, and peripheral vascular disease (PVD). Past surgical history (PSH) includes a right femoral popliteal bypass. On initial assessment at the clinic, a complete physical examination is done and reveals bruits on auscultation of the left carotid artery. An electrocardiogram (EKG) shows atrial fibrillation. Her vital signs are:

Blood pressure: 170/100

Pulse: 78 and irregular

Respirations: 20

Temperature: 98.4° F

Lab reports from the clinic reveal:

Prothrombin time (PT): 13.4 seconds, Control: 12.9 seconds

Partial thromboplastin time (PTT): 30 seconds, Control: 29.9 seconds

Glucose: 109 mg/dL

Blood urea nitrogen (BUN): 9 mg/dL

Creatinine: 0.8 mg/dL

Sodium (Na): 136 mEq/L

Potassium (K+): 3.9 mEq/L

Calcium: 9 mg/dL

Protein total: 7.8 g/dL

Albumin: 3.2 g/dL

Total bilirubin: 0.6

White blood cell (WBC) count: 10,300/mm^3

Red blood cell (RBC) count: 4.26 million/mm^3

Hemoglobin (Hgb): 11.7 g/dL

Hematocrit (Hct): 34.6%

Platelet count: 258,000/mm^3

Low-density lipoprotein (LDL): 127 mg/dL

High-density lipoprotein (HDL): 46 mg/dL

Total cholesterol: 257 mg/dL

Triglyceride: 220 mg/dL

Medications taken at home are brought to the clinic and include: simvastatin, felodipine, lisinopril, hydrochlorothiazide, and aspirin 325 mg (EC). Carotid duplex ultrasonography is done and reveals marked narrowing of proximal left external carotid artery with area of plaque noted. Her ejection fraction is 30%. Magnetic resonance imaging (MRI) is done and compared with carotid duplex ultrasonography; the results are similar. After a complete history and physical and review of serum labs and diagnostic studies, the diagnosis of atherosclerosis is confirmed. Ms. Z will be discharged to home and will return to the hospital as scheduled for possible carotid endarterectomy after reevaluation of current medication regimen and repeat carotid duplex ultrasonography. Ms. Z is referred to physical therapy for physical strengthening exercises.

The following are prescribed:

- Cholestyramine resin (Questran) 4 g PO four times per day, before meals
- Colestipol HcL (Colestid) 15 g two times per day, before meals and at bedtime
- Digoxin (Lanoxin) 0.125 mg PO daily
- Dipyridamole (Persantine) 75 mg PO four times per day
- Diltiazem HcL (Cardizem) 30 mg PO four times per day
- Warfarin sodium (Coumadin) 5 mg PO today

Questions

1. What are the most common cited coronary artery disease risk equivalents for atherosclerosis?

2. What are the prominent modifiable and non-modifiable risk factors of atheroslcerosis?

3. What are common nursing diagnoses for the client with atherosclerosis?

4. What are the purposes for the prescribed medications?

5. What are the most common adverse reactions of the prescribed medications?

6. Discuss the drug-to-drug and drug-to-food/herbal interactions of the prescribed medications.

7. What are some physical findings in carotid stenosis?

8. What are some psychosocial stressors that can worsen hypertension and affect the client's ability to collaborate with treatment?

9. If Ms. Z is noncompliant with medical regimen after discharge and develops hypertensive crisis and is brought to the emergency department (ED), what are the indicators the nurse should focus on eliciting from the client on initial contact?

10. How should the nurse discuss discharge plans with Ms. Z in regard to her admission weight, at 5'5", of 248 pounds?

CASE STUDY 3

Chronic Vascular Ulcers of the Right Foot

GENDER

M

AGE

78

SETTING

- Hospital

ETHNICITY/CULTURE

- Black American

PREEXISTING CONDITIONS

- Diabetes
- Hypertension

COEXISTING CONDITIONS

- Coronary artery bypass stroke
- Stroke

LIFESTYLE

- Retired

COMMUNICATION

DISABILITY

- Immobility

SOCIOECONOMIC STATUS

- Middle

SPIRITUAL/RELIGIOUS

- Baptist

PHARMACOLOGIC

- Rosiglitazone maleate (Avandia)
- Ticarcillin disodium/clavulanate potassium (Timentin)
- Gentamicin sulfate (Garamycin)
- Gabapentin (Neurontin)
- Enoxaparin (Lovenox)

PSYCHOSOCIAL

- Anxiety

LEGAL

ETHICAL

ALTERNATIVE THERAPY

Prayer

PRIORITIZATION

- Microbiological control
- Metabolic control
- Vascular control
- Wound control

DELEGATION

- RN
- Wound care specialist
- CNA

THE CARDIOVASCULAR AND LYMPHATIC SYSTEMS

Level of difficulty: Moderate

Overview: This case involves accurate identification of weak or absent peripheral pulses; sensation of bilateral extremities; pain on toes, between toes, and on upper aspect of the foot. Critical-thinking skills are used to prioritize effective care.

Client Profile

Mr. M is a 78-year-old retired lieutenant of the U.S. Army. He is 5'10" and weighs 190 pounds. He is admitted from a nursing home with ulcers on the right great toe and plantar surface of the right foot.

Case Study

On admission to the hospital, Mr. M's vital signs are:

Blood pressure: 170/98

Pulse: 76

Respirations: 20

Temperature: 100.9° F

He is alert and oriented to time, place, and person. He has an indwelling Foley catheter in place to straight drainage, which is draining amber-colored urine. The following lab reports are sent from the nursing home:

White blood cell (WBC) count: 18,000/mm^3

Red blood cell (RBC) count: 3,000,000/uL

Hemoglobin (Hgb): 16.4 g/dL

Hematocrit (Hct): 34%

Platelet count (PLT): 298,000/mm^3

Glucose: 208 mg/dL

Blood urea nitrogen (BUN): 12 mg/dL

Past medical history (PMH) includes type 2 diabetes mellitus (non-independent diabetes mellitus [NIDDM]), peripheral vascular disease (PVD), hypertension, benign prostatic hyperplasia (BPH), depression, status-post (S/P) cerebrovascular accident (CVA) two years ago. Past surgical history (PSH) includes status-post (S/P) coronary artery bypass graft (CABG) and S/P femoral popliteal bypass and femoral endarterectomy one year ago. Medications sent with certified nursing assistant (CNA) who accompanied him to the hospital include: fluoxetine HcL, aspirin EC, ferrous sulfate, folic acid, gemfibrozil, finasteride, furosemide, metoprolol tartrate, omeprazole, and rosiglitazone maleate. Plans to review the medications brought to the hospital at a later time and renew them as appropriate are discussed by the health care provider and the primary nurse, the wound care specialist, and a pharmacist. Blood and wound culture is done and reveals Pseudomonas aeruginosa. The health care provider does a history and physical including a head-to-toe assessment. During the assessment of the lower extremities, the client reports pain in the lower right extremity during ambulation and at rest. Bilateral lower extremities are thoroughly assessed for color, temperature, pulses, odor, or drainage from the ulcer. An ankle brachial index (ABI) is done on both extremities and reveals an ABI 0.6 of the right lower extremity and a 0.9 of the left lower extremity. A surgical consult is requested and done, and the health care provider orders a duplex ultrasonography with color flow Doppler that shows chronic ischemic areas of the foot. After the multidisciplinary team reviews the labs and diagnostic reports, a medical diagnosis of vascular ulcers of the right foot is made. A discussion with Mr. M is done pertaining to management of the wound. Surgical débridement is discussed, and informed consent witnessed and signed by Mr. M. The débridement is scheduled for the next day. The débridement is successful. The client returns from the surgical procedure with an intact transparent wound barrier dressing to the foot and a vacuum-assisted pump applied with negative pressure to the ulcer area.

The following are prescribed:

- Morphine sulfate (Duramorph) 8 mg IM q4h PRN pain × 3 days
- Ticarcillin disodium/clavulanate potassium (Timentin) 3.1 g q6h
- Rosiglitazone maleate (Avandia) 8 mg PO daily
- Metoprolol tartrate (Lopressor) 75 mg PO daily
- Furosemide (Lasix) 49 mg PO daily
- Gabapentin (Neurontin) 400 mg PO q8h
- Enoxaparin (Lovenox) 30 mg/0.3 ML SC q12h
- Oxycodone/acetaminophen (Endocet) 5/325 MG 2 tablets PO q4h PRN
- Fingerstick glucose every shift and PRN
- Serum labs: glucose, WBC

Questions

1. Discuss risk factors and pathophysiology of vascular ulcers of the lower extremities.

2. Discuss the clinical manifestations for vascular disease of the lower extremities.

3. Discuss diagnostic studies used to confirm the diagnosis of vascular ulcers of the lower extremities.

4. Discuss common nursing diagnoses for vascular ulcers of the lower extremities.

5. What are the purposes for the prescribed orders?

6. What are the most common adverse reactions, drug-to-drug, drug-to-food/herbal interactions for the prescribed medications?

7. Discuss surgical management for peripheral artery disease of the lower extremities.

8. Discuss client education for vascular ulcers of the lower extremities.

Disseminated Intravascular Coagulation

GENDER

F

AGE

56

SETTING

■ Hospital

ETHNICITY/CULTURE

■ Black American

PREEXISTING CONDITIONS

■ History of intestinal obstruction

COEXISTING CONDITIONS

LIFESTYLE

■ Health educator who lectures four days per week at a senior college

COMMUNICATION

DISABILITY

SOCIOECONOMIC STATUS

■ Middle

SPIRITUAL/RELIGIOUS

■ Evangelical

PHARMACOLOGIC

■ Gentamicin sulfate (Garamycin)
■ Clindamycin HcL (Cleocin Hydrochloride)
■ Cryoprecipitate
■ Aminocaproic acid
■ Vancomycin HcL (Vancocin)
■ Metronidazole (Flagyl)

PSYCHOSOCIAL

■ Anxiety
■ Pain

LEGAL

ETHICAL

■ The right to make decisions related to care

ALTERNATIVE THERAPY

■ Prayer

PRIORITIZATION

■ Patent airway
■ Improve circulatory volume
■ Supportive therapy with blood components

DELEGATION

■ RN
■ Client education

MODERATE

THE CARDIOVASCULAR AND LYMPHATIC SYSTEMS

Level of difficulty: Moderate

Overview: The case involves critical-thinking skills to prioritize and delegate care efficiently and appropriately. It involves clinical expertise in caring for the client with potential for thrombi and bleeding, and acute renal failure (ARF). It requires a multidisciplinary team with a clear understanding of the physiological changes that occur in disseminated intravascular coagulation.

Client Profile

Mrs. L is a 56-year-old female who for the past month has experienced occasional nausea and dizziness. After returning home from her teaching assignment, Mrs. L experienced a moderately sharp pain across her umbilicus. She had a cup of tea then went to rest and fell asleep. Upon awakening, Mrs. L experienced a more severe, intolerable pain of the abdomen. She is accompanied by a neighbor to her family health care provider and, on arrival at the health care provider's office, is immediately transferred to the emergency department (ED) of a nearby hospital.

Case Study

In the ED, a quick systems assessment is done followed by an upper gastrointestinal radiographic series (UGIS), which is ineffective because she vomits contents of the barium sulfate, including fecal content seen in the vomitus. Mrs. L is transferred to a surgical unit, and a systematic approach is used in doing the nursing history. Serum, urine specimens, and blood cultures are collected and sent to the laboratory. A chest X-ray, abdominal X-ray, and electrocardiogram (EKG) are completed, and the informed consent is signed. The abdominal X-ray reveals large amounts of fecal contents resting in the small intestines. Mrs. L's husband is notified of the plans for surgery, and Mrs. L is prepared for emergency laparotomy. A nasogastric tube (NGT) is inserted and attached to low continuous suction, and a Foley catheter is inserted and placed to straight drainage. Mrs. L is transferred to the operating room (OR) with a tentative diagnosis of mechanical obstruction of the small intestines. The initial surgery is successful and Mrs. L is returned to the surgical unit. On arrival, there is gentamicin 80 mg IV, Ringers Lactate at 125 cc/hr, morphine sulfate via PCA at 1 mg continuous, 5 mg PCA dose every eight minutes, and Foley catheter draining amber-colored urine at 50cc/hr. Mrs. L is drowsy but responsive to name and painful stimuli. Vital signs are:

> Blood pressure: 130/80
>
> Pulse: 100
>
> Respirations: 16
>
> Temperature: 98.0° F

On post-op day one, a consultation is written for an infectious disease health care provider to approve intravenous clindamycin due to the large strains of gram-positive cocci, including E. coli and C. difficle, which were cultured from fecal contents of the intestines. Clindamycin 1500 mg is prescribed and is started on post-op day two. Within minutes after clindamycin is started, Mrs. L develops large wheals over her entire body, with pustules over the face and upper and lower extremities, and profuse watery diarrhea. Clindamycin is immediately discontinued and intravenous diphenhydramine HcL is administered. Ceftriaxone sodium IV is initiated. Mrs. L's condition worsens with evidence of high fever of 106.6° F, shaking chills, B/P 90/60, respirations 24, and pulse 120. She is immediately transferred to the surgical intensive care unit and is placed on four liters of oxygen via nasal cannula and 0.9% NaCL initiated at 150 mL/hr. Continuous monitoring of oxygen saturation with pulse oximeter, frequent arterial blood gases (ABGs), and accurate urinary output from indwelling catheter are maintained. On post-op day three, her condition deteriorates and a tentative diagnosis of sepsis-induced distributive shock is made. Laboratory data reveal:

> Fibrinogen level: 200 mg/dL
>
> D-dimer: 150 ng/mL

Bleeding time: 20 minutes

Platelet count (PLT): 100,000/mm³

Prothrombin time (PT) with INR: 3.8

Activated partial thromboplastin time (aPTT): 80 seconds

Partial thromboplastin time (PTT): 90 seconds

White blood cell (WBC) count: 20,000/mm³

After the labs are reviewed, a diagnosis of disseminated intravascular coagulation (DIC) secondary to sepsis-induced distributive shock is made.

The following are prescribed:

- Gentamicin sulfate (Garamycin) 2 mg/kg IV stat, followed by 3 mg/kg IV q8h
- Clindamycin HcL (Cleocin Hydrochloride) 1,500 mg q6h IV
- Metronidazole (Flagyl) 7.5 mg/kg q6h IV
- Diphenhydramine HcL (Benadryl) 50 mg IV stat
- Ceftriaxone sodium (Rocephin) 2 g q12h IV
- Fresh frozen plasma 1 unit IV
- Drotrecogin alfa (Activated) (Xigris) 24 mcg/kg/h continuous infusion × 96 h
- Daily serum labs: fibrinogen, D-dimer, bleeding time, PLT, PT, PTT

Questions

1. Discuss some specific factors that cause DIC.

2. Discuss common nursing diagnoses for clients with DIC.

3. What was the main purpose for the NGT to suction while the client was in the ED?

4. What is the reason for withholding opioid analgesic from Mrs. L, even though she is complaining of severe abdominal pain on arrival to the ED?

5. What are the purposes for the prescribed medications post-surgery?

6. If the client has developed anaphylaxis due to adverse reaction to the clindamycin, what reversal agent would most likely be prescribed?

7. What are the most common adverse reactions of the prescribed medications?

8. Why are the specified serum labs ordered for Mrs. L?

9. Discuss the drug-to-drug and drug-to-food/herbal interactions for the prescribed medications.

10. What is an important reminder for Mrs. L prior to her discharge?

11. You are a community-based nurse for a visiting nurse service. You are assigned to supervise home-care management in preparation for Mrs. L to return home upon discharge. A home health aide (HHA) is assigned to Mrs. L's care, with RN visits five days per week for the first week, three days per week for the second week, and one day per week for two additional weeks. Develop a community-based plan of care for the HHA to follow in the absence of the RN.

Unstable Angina Pectoris (Acute Myocardial Ischemia)

GENDER

F

AGE

60

SETTING

- Hospital

ETHNICITY/CULTURE

- Hispanic American

PREEXISTING CONDITIONS

- Atherosclerosis
- Coronary spasms
- Anemia

COEXISTING CONDITIONS

- Hyperthyroidism
- Stimulant abuse

LIFESTYLE

- Accounting department supervisor

COMMUNICATION

- Spanish and English

DISABILITY

SOCIOECONOMIC STATUS

- Middle

SPIRITUAL/RELIGIOUS

- Nondenominational

PHARMACOLOGIC

- Nitrates
- Beta-adrenergic blockers
- Calcium-channel blockers
- Aspirin

PSYCHOSOCIAL

- Anxiety

LEGAL

ETHICAL

ALTERNATIVE THERAPY

- Acupuncture
- Ginseng

PRIORITIZATION

- Obtain description of client's chest discomfort
- Obtain 12-lead EKG
- Provide measures to enhance tissue perfusion

DELEGATION

- RN
- Client education

MODERATE

THE CARDIOVASCULAR AND LYMPHATIC SYSTEMS

Level of difficulty: Moderate

Overview: This case involves a thorough assessment and critical-thinking skills to identify the classic symptoms of unstable angina so that appropriate medical interventions can be implemented effectively and to prioritize clients, because clients with unstable angina can progress to myocardial infarction or even death.

Client Profile

Ms. T, a 60-year-old female, is brought to the hospital emergency department (ED) due to intolerable chest pain after climbing several flights of stairs at her place of employment. Ms. T is 5′5″ and weighs 206 pounds. Ms. T is an accounting department supervisor. She is a good historian and is able to explain quality and intensity of the present symptoms that warranted her access to the hospital ED.

Case Study

Ms. T reports taking nitroglycerin (NTG) for chest pain but says she did not take her NTG tablets to work with her, therefore, the pain was worse than she had experienced with previous attacks. However, on arrival to the ED, she reports that the severity of the pain has subsided. Ms. T's vital signs on arrival to the ED are:

> Blood pressure: 118/84
>
> Pulse: 74 and irregular
>
> Respirations: 22
>
> Temperature: 98.2° F

A 12-lead electrocardiogram (EKG) is done and reveals ST depression, T-wave inversion, atrioventricular conduction delay, and atrial fibrillation. Ms. T presently denies any discomfort and is waiting to be seen by the nurse practitioner (NP). The NP in the ED is given the report of the 12-lead EKG and will collaborate with the health care provider. As the interview with the NP continues, Ms. T reports inability to walk more than two blocks without difficulty breathing. She further reports noticing these occurrences increasing over the past three weeks. Her past medical history (PMH) includes aortic stenosis and hyperlipidemia and a right- and left-heart catheterization seven years ago. She reports being monitored in a cardiology clinic by a team of cardiologists. Reports from her medical records indicate moderate stenosis of the left anterior descending (LAD) artery. She has mild pulmonary hypertension, mild coronary atherosclerosis, and a mildly increased left ventricular hypertrophy. Her right coronary artery (RCA) shows mild calcification, and the LAD and the circumflex artery have moderate lesions. She is admitted to the coronary care unit (CCU), and continuous telemetry is initiated. The health care provider prescribes an echocardiogram and exercise stress test. The findings are positive for myocardial ischemia with decreased ejection fraction noted. Current laboratory values reveal:

> White blood cell (WBC) count: 10,000/mm^3
>
> CK-MB: 132 U/L
>
> Hematocrit (Hct): 32%
>
> Hemoglobin (Hgb): 12 g/dL
>
> Potassium (K+): 4 mEq/L
>
> Sodium (Na): 145 mEq/L
>
> Troponin: T_1 0.1 ng/mL
>
> LDH_1: 38%
>
> LDH_2: 40%
>
> Total serum cholesterol: 185 mg/dL
>
> Triglyceride: 165 mg/dL

After review of diagnostic studies, laboratory data, physical assessment, and client's subjective data, a diagnosis of unstable angina pectoris is made. The health care team decides that Ms. T can return home, with follow-up care with her primary health care provider within two weeks from today's date. A repeat 12-lead EKG is done without any changes noted from the initial one. Ms. T is resting and her vital signs are:

Blood pressure: 118/78

Pulse: 74 irregular

Respirations: 18

Temperature: 98.2° F

The cardiologist and the NP discuss the discharge criteria with Ms. T, and she is to be discharged within 24 hours. The social worker and registered dietitian will visit with Ms. T in preparation for discharge.

The following are prescribed at discharge:

- Nitroglycerin (NTG) tab 0.4 mg SL for chest pain PRN
- Propranolol HcL (Inderal) 40 mg PO two times per day
- Nifedipine (Procardia) 20 mg PO three times per day
- Clopidogrel bisulfate (Plavix) 75 mg PO daily

Questions

1. What is your understanding of the above situation?

2. What is the incidence according to the American Heart Association (AHA) in regard to being overweight and obesity?

3. Discuss the relationship between gender and acute coronary syndrome (angina).

4. Explain the two predominant types of angina.

5. Discuss common nursing diagnoses for clients with angina pectoris.

6. If the following diagnostic tests were ordered for Ms. T, what would be the expected results?

- Chest radiography
- Echocardiogram

7. When would surgical intervention be considered for Ms. T?

8. What are the purposes for the prescribed medications?

9. What are the most common adverse reactions of the prescribed medications?

10. Discuss the drug-to-drug and drug-to-food/herbal interactions for the prescribed medications.

11. Discuss client education for unstable angina and aortic stenosis.

Sternal Wound Infection

GENDER

M

AGE

66

SETTING

- Hospital

ETHNICITY/CULTURE

- White American

PREEXISTING CONDITIONS

COEXISTING CONDITIONS

- Coronary artery bypass graft

LIFESTYLE

- Self-employed construction worker

COMMUNICATION

DISABILITY

SOCIOECONOMIC STATUS

- Middle

SPIRITUAL/RELIGIOUS

- Catholic

PHARMACOLOGIC

- Morphine sulfate (Duramorph)
- Piperacillin sodium/Tazobactam sodium (Zosyn)
- Ciprofloxacin HcL (Cipro)

PSYCHOSOCIAL

- Anxiety

LEGAL

ETHICAL

- Quality care
- Decrease in income
- Health care benefits

ALTERNATIVE THERAPY

- St. John's Wort

PRIORITIZATION

- Room assignment
- Antimicrobial management

DELEGATION

- RN
- Wound care specialist
- CNA

MODERATE

THE CARDIOVASCULAR AND LYMPHATIC SYSTEMS

Level of difficulty: Moderate

Overview: This case focuses on the use of critical thinking to provide effective prioritization in a triage situation in a busy urban medical center emergency department. It also involves management of sternal wound infection secondary to post-coronary artery bypass graft. A wound care specialist is important to management of an infected wound. The certified nursing assistant (CNA) can help with assembling necessary equipment in preparation for wound care and can position the client for the performance of the wound care.

Client Profile

Mr. Y is a 66-year-old male who was discharged from the hospital six weeks ago after an emergency quadruple coronary artery bypass graft (CABG) surgery. His post-op recovery was uneventful, and he was discharged ten days after the surgery. He returns to the chief surgeon's private office on the tenth day post-discharge prior to readmission because the sternal incisional site is red and inflamed with an unusual odor from the site of the wound. He reports pain at the site during hygiene care and a temperature of 101.2° F during the five days prior to seeing the health care provider. Mr. Y believes the redness at the incisional site is normal after surgery. However, because of the unusual odor, he goes to the health care provider's office to have the wound evaluated. Mr. Y is 5′8″ and weighs 206 pounds.

Case Study

Mr. Y is referred to the hospital for further evaluation. On initial interview his vital signs are:

> Blood pressure: 130/84
> Pulse: 78 and regular
> Respirations: 20
> Temperature: 102.4° F

The sternal incision is red, raised, and moderately warm to touch. There are no signs of dehiscence although the wound edges are not completely approximated. Mr. Y reports a 30-year history of cigarette smoking, three packs per week. His past medical history (PMH) includes hyperlipidemia, stable angina, and past surgical history of left cardiac catheterization and percutaneous transluminal coronary angioplasty (PTCA) with stent two years ago. Lab test results sent from the health care provider's office reveal:

> White blood cell (WBC) count: 12,000/mm^3
> Red blood cell (RBC) count: 4.6/mm^3
> Calcium: 9 mg/dL
> Sodium (Na): 142 mEq/L
> Potassium (K+): 4.9 mEq/L
> Chloride: 100 mEq/L
> Blood urea nitrogen (BUN): 15 mg/dL
> Creatinine: 1.4 mg/dL
> Glucose: 130 mg/dL
> Platelet count (PLT): 300, 000/cm
> Prothrombin time (PT): 14 seconds, Control: 15.1 seconds
> Hematocrit (Hct): 42%
> Hemoglobin (Hgb): 16 g/dL
> Low-density lipoprotein (LDL): 130 mg/dL
> Total cholesterol: 200 mg/dL

Medications brought to the hospital include: lovastatin (Mevacor), nitroglycerin (NTG) sublingual, isosorbide dinitrate (Isordil), warfarin sodium (Coumadin) 7.5 mg, and rabeprazole sodium (Aciphex). Mr. Y is transferred to a cardio-thoracic unit. A computed tomography (CT) scan of the chest is done in the ED and there is no evidence of infection in the deeper structures of the thoracic cavity.

On continued interview, Mr. Y reports self-medication with St. John's Wort whenever he feels anxious. His sternal wound is inspected by the receiving nurse who documents and reports the finding. Wound specimen for culture and sensitivity, and blood for gram stain are done and sent to the lab. An electrocardiogram (EKG) and a chest X-ray are done upon arrival to the unit, nursing assessment is completed, Mr. Y is placed on telemetry, and the nurse documents assessment findings. A nurse practitioner (NP) reviews the medications with the client and will discuss with the cardiologist before including them in current orders. The lab sends the report of the cultures, and the results are positive for Staphylococcus aureus and Enterococcus species. Mr. Y is informed that he will be admitted for further evaluation and antibiotic therapy. A diagnosis of sternal wound infection is made.

The following are prescribed:

- Piperacillin sodium/tazobactam sodium (Zosyn) 3 g IV q8h
- Morphine sulfate (Duramorph) PRN 2 mg IV prior to each dressing change
- Oxycodone (Roxicodone) 5–10 mg q4h PRN for mild to moderate pain
- Lovastatin (Mevacor) 40 mg PO two times per day
- Isosorbide dinitrate (Isordil) 10 mg four times per day PO, before meals and at bedtime
- Rabeprazole sodium (Aciphex) 20 mg PO daily
- Warfarin sodium (Coumadin) 7.5 mg PO daily after checking PT level
- Wound irrigation with 0.9% normal saline solution two times per day, followed by a wet-to-moist packing with 0.9% normal saline solution

Questions

1. What is a local factor that has affected Mr. Y's wound healing?

2. How do age, chronic disease, and vascular problems delay Mr. Y's wound healing?

3. Discuss common nursing diagnoses related to wound management.

4. What are the purposes for the prescribed medications?

5. What are the most common adverse reactions of the prescribed medications?

6. Discuss the drug-to-drug and drug-to-food/herbal interactions of the prescribed medications.

7. How do drugs such as corticosteroids, anti-inflammatory agents, and chemotherapy delay wound healing?

8. How do years of cigarette smoking delay wound healing?

9. What are the benefits of wound irrigation?

10. Discuss the phases of wound healing.

11. Discuss client education at time of discharge for an unhealed wound.

CASE STUDY 7

Valvular Heart Disease – Aortic Stenosis

GENDER

M

AGE

56

SETTING

■ Hospital

ETHNICITY/CULTURE

■ Hispanic/American

PREEXISTING CONDITIONS

■ Angina

COEXISTING CONDITIONS

LIFESTYLE

■ Supervisor for a community department store

COMMUNICATION

■ Spanish and English

DISABILITY

SOCIOECONOMIC STATUS

■ Middle

SPIRITUAL/RELIGIOUS

■ Catholic

PHARMACOLOGIC

■ Calcium-channel blocker
■ ACE inhibitor
■ Cardiotonic
■ Oxygen

PSYCHOSOCIAL

■ Anxiety

LEGAL

ETHICAL

ALTERNATIVE THERAPY

■ Holy Communion

PRIORITIZATION

■ Maintain cardiac output
■ Monitor vital signs
■ Administer oxygen

DELEGATION

■ RN
■ Client education

THE CARDIOVASCULAR AND LYMPHATIC SYSTEMS

Level of difficulty: Moderate

Overview: This case involves the use of the nursing process and critical thinking to appropriately assess the client and delegate effectively so that care can be implemented. The case requires health care personnel who are competent in cardiac assessment, identifying heart sounds and dysrhythmias, and intervening effectively.

Client Profile

Mr. W is a 56-year-old male who is 5′6″ and weighs 190 pounds. His past medical history includes childhood rheumatic heart disease with one occurrence of strep throat at the age of 30. Mr. W is married, and there is one young adult living at home with him and his wife. They live in a private home with four flights of steps going up to the bedrooms.

Case Study

Mr. W is referred to the hospital by his primary health care provider after frequent complaints of difficulty breathing when climbing stairs and a report of feeling tired after walking only two blocks. Mr. W also reports anginal-type chest pain and infrequent syncope. He reports loss of appetite and loss of 12 pounds over one month. On admission to the hospital, his vitals signs are:

Blood pressure: 150/68

Pulse: 64 and irregular

Respirations: 16

Temperature: 98.6° F

On auscultation, there is a harsh systolic murmur in the second intercostal space at the right sternal border. An arterial blood gas (ABG) is done and reveals hypoxemia. Oxygen, three liters via nasal cannula, is initiated. Mr. W denies surgical history but reports having a cardiac catheterization that was done two months ago at another hospital and chronic atrial fibrillation. The result of the catheterization is sent from Mr. W's primary health care provider's office. The report of the catheterization is:

Routine blood pressure in brachial artery: 120/50 mm Hg
  (normal = 90–140/60–90 mm Hg)

End-diastolic volume (EDV): 80 ml/m² (normal = 50–90 ml/m²)

Ejection fraction: 0.58 (normal = 0.67 ± 0.07)

Cardiac output: (CO) 4 liters/min (normal = 3–6 liters/min)

A thorough history and physical is completed by a health care provider and a registered nurse (RN). A multidisciplinary team reviews the current data gathered from the history, physical, and reports of the previous diagnostic tests. A chest X-ray reveals mid-left ventricular enlargement, and echocardiography provides data of the cardiac structure, movement of the valve leaflets, and the size and function of the cardiac chambers, which aids in diagnosis. An EKG confirms chronic atrial fibrillation. Admission lab tests reveal:

White blood cell (WBC) count: 9,000/mm³

Red blood cell (RBC): 3.4 million/mm³

Hemoglobin (Hgb): 10 g/dL

Hematocrit (Hct): 28%

Platelet: 150,000/mm³

Glucose: 116 mg/dL

Blood urea nitrogen (BUN): 15 mg/dL

Creatinine: 0.9 mg/dL

Sodium (Na): 135 mEq/L

Potassium (K+): 4.6 mEq/L

Albumin: 3.3 mg/dL

Calcium: 8.6 mg/dL

Digoxin level: 1.3 ng/dL

After review of collected data and collaborative discussion with the multidisciplinary team, a diagnosis of aortic stenosis is confirmed. The findings are discussed with Mr. W and his wife, and a surgical consultation is done. Elective surgery for aortic valve repair is planned and will be scheduled within three days. A prosthetic valve will be used. In preparation for the aortic valve repair, Mr. W is to be transfused as prescribed with two units of packed red blood cells (PRBCs) because of the low Hgb and Hct.

The following new medications are prescribed:

- Digoxin (Lanoxin) 0.125 mg PO
- Diltiazem (Cardizem) 40 mg PO two times per day
- Amiodarone HcL (Cardarone) 200 mg PO daily
- Warfarin sodium (Coumadin) 5 mg PO today

Questions

1. Discuss common nursing diagnoses for clients with valvular heart disease.

2. Why is cardiac catheterization usually done when clients are diagnosed with aortic stenosis?

3. Why is atrial fibrillation a common finding in aortic stenosis?

4. What is a long-term complication of aortic stenosis?

5. What are the purposes for the prescribed orders?

6. What are the most common adverse reactions of the prescribed medications?

7. Discuss the drug-to-drug and drug-to-food/herbal interactions of the prescribed medications.

8. Which modality is the definitive treatment of aortic stenosis for clients with complaints of dyspnea, fatigue, and chest pain?

9. Identify the different types of valves used in valvular replacement procedures.

10. What are the two post-surgery complications the nurse should monitor for when a client has a valvular replacement?

11. Discuss client education for post-valvular surgery?

CASE STUDY 8

Hodgkin's Disease

GENDER

M

AGE

54

SETTING

- Outpatient clinic of a medical center

ETHNICITY/CULTURE

- White Englishman

PREEXISTING CONDITIONS

- Enlarged, painless, freely movable mass in the neck

COEXISTING CONDITIONS

- History of viral infection

LIFESTYLE

- Worked as a subway worker before immigrating to the U.S.

COMMUNICATION

DISABILITY

SOCIOECONOMIC STATUS

- Middle

SPIRITUAL/RELIGIOUS

- Anglican

PHARMACOLOGIC

- Mechlorethamine HcL (Mustargen)
- Vincristine sulfate (Oncovin)
- Procarbazine HcL (Matulane)
- Prednisone (Deltasone)
- Ondansetron HcL (Zofran)

PSYCHOSOCIAL

- Anxiety

LEGAL

- Assistance with financial resource

ETHICAL

- Do recent immigrants to the U.S. have a right to optimum health care benefits in lieu of unemployment related to work status?

ALTERNATIVE THERAPY

PRIORITIZATION

- Physical assessment
- Prepare for staging of lymph node

DELEGATION

- RN
- Client education

THE CARDIOVASCULAR AND LYMPHATIC SYSTEMS

Level of difficulty: Moderate

Overview: This case study involves a thorough assessment of the client's condition with careful palpation for lymphadenopathic lesions. It also involves critical questioning pertaining to night sweats and weight loss of more than 10%, unusual headaches, dry cough, and neck or back pain.

Client Profile

Mr. O is a 54-year-old male who has been a resident of the United States for the past three years after relocating from London, England, where he worked as an underground railroad employee. He is 5′8″ and weighs 165 pounds.

Case Study

Mr. O is seen in the outpatient clinic of a major medical center with complaints of gradual fatigue and weight loss over the past two months. He also reports fever of unknown cause, unusual pruritus on the trunk and chest of his body, headaches, and vertigo. After initial interview by the nurse, Mr. O is seen by a health care provider, who continues with the history and physical examination. Large, painless lymph nodes are found in the neck and axilla areas. Mr. O denies the use of medications or herbal supplements and denies past medical or surgical history. Vital signs on admission reveal:

> Blood pressure: 120/80
>
> Pulse: 78
>
> Respirations: 16
>
> Temperature: 98.4° F

Lab results reveal:

> White blood cell (WBC) differential:
>> Lymphocytes: 22%
>>
>> Segmented neutrophils: 60%
>>
>> Monocytes: 6.2%
>>
>> Eosinophils: 0.9%
>>
>> Basophils: 1.1%
>>
>> Bands: 5%
>
> Red blood cell (RBC) count: 4 million/mm^3
>
> Hematocrit (Hct): 42%
>
> Hemoglobin (Hgb): 13 g/dL
>
> Platelet count: 267,000/mm^3
>
> Granulocyte: 20.4%
>
> Sodium (Na): 138 mEq/L
>
> Potassium (K+): 3.9 mEq/L
>
> Calcium: 8.4 mg/dL
>
> Blood urea nitrogen (BUN): 15 mg/dL
>
> Creatinine: 0.7 mg/dL
>
> Magnesium: 2 mg/dL

After the labs and physical assessment findings are reviewed by the health care provider and a hematologist, Mr. O is admitted to a medical unit for further evaluation. A positron emission test (PET) shows cancer cells in the peripheral lymph node and peripheral lymph node enlargement. A chest X-ray and an abdominal computed tomography (CT) scan are done, but the findings for lymphadenopathy in the thoracic and abdominal areas are negative. Mr. O is advised of the need for lymph node biopsy, and he signs an informed witnessed consent. The biopsy is positive for Reed-Sternberg cells. Staging procedures reveal stage IIa lymphoma. After the health care provider and hematologist review the results of the labs and diagnostic reports, a diagnosis of stage IIa Hodgkin's disease is confirmed and discussed with the client, who agrees with the treatment plan.

The following are prescribed:

- MOPP combination therapy q4 weeks for six cycles:
- Mechlorethamine HcL (Mustargen) IV 6 mg/m^2 on day one and eight of a 28-day cycle
- Vincristine sulfate (Oncovin) IV 1.4 mg/m^2 weekly
- Procarbazine HcL (Matulane) PO 2 mg/kg/d for one week, then 6 mg/kg/d
- Prednisone (Deltasone) 30 mg PO daily
- Ondansetron HcL (Zofran) 32 mg IV 30 minutes before chemotherapy

Questions

1. Discuss the prevalence, incidence, risk factors, and pathophysiology of Hodgkin's disease.

2. Discuss clinical manifestations of Hodgkin's disease.

3. Discuss diagnostic studies used to confirm Hodgkin's disease.

4. Discuss medical management for Hodgkin's disease.

5. Discuss complications of Hodgkin's disease.

6. What are the purposes for the prescribed medications?

7. What are the most common adverse reactions, drug-to-drug, drug-to-food/herbal interactions of the prescribed mediations?

8. Discuss staging classification for Hodgkin's disease.

9. Discuss management for vincristine infusion therapy.

10. Discuss client education for Hodgkin's disease.

CASE STUDY 9

Multiple Myeloma (Plasma Cell Myeloma)

GENDER

F

AGE

64

SETTING

- Hospital

ETHNICITY/CULTURE

- Black American

PREEXISTING CONDITIONS

COEXISTING CONDITIONS

- Renal failure

LIFESTYLE

- Worked 15 years for a company that sells wood and soil for agricultural and building purposes

COMMUNICATION

DISABILITY

- Difficulty ambulating independently

SOCIOECONOMIC STATUS

- Middle

SPIRITUAL/RELIGIOUS

- Baptist

PHARMACOLOGIC

- Acetaminophen (Tylenol)
- Melphalan (Alkeran)
- Prednisone (Deltasone)
- Pamidronate disodium (Aredia)
- Cyclophosphamide (Cytoxan)
- Furosemide (Lasix)
- Palonosetron HcL (Aloxi)

PSYCHOSOCIAL

- Anxiety

LEGAL

- Supplemental resource to defray hospital expenses

ETHICAL

- The right to receive disability benefits if illness is job related

ALTERNATIVE THERAPY

- Fish oil

PRIORITIZATION

- Assess bone or joint pain
- Promote comfort
- Provide safety

DELEGATION

- RN
- CNA
- Client education

THE CARDIOVASCULAR AND LYMPHATIC SYSTEMS

Level of difficulty: Moderate

Overview: This case involves a thorough assessment of the client's condition with focus on bone and joint pain, easy bruising, and signs of renal insufficiency. It involves nursing measures to avoid exposure to infections. The certified nursing assistant (CNA) can be delegated the duty of observing for discoloration while assisting with hygiene care.

Client Profile

Mrs. R, a 64-year-old widow for the past ten years, is accompanied by her home health aide (HHA) via ambulance to the hospital's emergency department (ED) after falling at home. Mrs. R is 4′5″ and weighs 120 pounds.

Case Study

On arrival in the triage area, she reports pain of the right upper extremity, which she said began after she fell at home. The nurse attempts to assess the upper extremity but is unable to do so because of the pain and the guarding of the extremity by Mrs. R. On initial interview, she reports being fatigued, weak, anorexic, and constipated for the past four days. She describes back and joint pain that is not related to her recent fall and explains that the pain is worse in the supine position and is not relieved by ibuprofen or acetaminophen. Mrs. R points to bluish discoloration on areas of her body, which she believes occur whenever she bumps on an object in her apartment. The HHA confirms the report of easy bruising, telling the nurse that Mrs. R bruises even with the slightest contact on soft furniture, and informs the nurse that Mrs. R has been showing signs of confusion and occasional disorientation for the past two weeks. Mrs. R denies significant past medical history but reports fracture of the left ankle that occurred six months ago due to a fall while ambulating in her apartment. Mrs. R is seen by the health care provider and a history and physical are done. She is then admitted to a medical unit for further evaluation and diagnosis. Serum lab reports reveal:

Calcium: 16.5 mg/dL

Phosphorous: 2.5 mg/dL

Neutrophils: 2,500%

Lymphocytes: 2,000/mm³

Monocytes: 150/mm³

Eosinophils: 200/mm³

Basophils: 80/mm³

Red blood cell (RBC) count: 4.2 mm³

Platelet count: 140,000 cells/mm³

Creatinine: 1.5 mg/dL

Blood urea nitrogen (BUN): 9 mg/dL

A bone marrow biopsy is done, after an informed consent is signed, and shows significant presence of sheets of malignant plasma cells. A 24-hour urinalysis by protein electrophoresis is positive for Bence Jones protein, and X-ray studies of bones find thinning and signs of osteoporosis and osteopenia. A diagnosis of multiple myeloma is confirmed.

The following are prescribed:
- Cyclophosphamide (Cytoxen) 10 mg/kg IV once daily × five days
- M combined with elphalan (Alkeran) 9 mg/PO daily × four days; alternate with 6 mg PO daily × seven days
- Prednisone (Deltasone) 50 mg PO two times per day × four days; alternate with 100 mg PO daily × seven days
- Pamidronate disodium (Aredia) 30 mg once daily IV × three days
- Palonosetron HcL (Aloxi) 0.25 mg IV 30 minutes before administration of antineoplastic

- Monitor serum labs daily: WBC count, Hct, Hgb, leukocytes, PLT, calcium, creatinine, BUN, and phosphorous
- Monitor urine for blood each void
- Maintain fluid hydration 3,000 mL daily and monitor intake and output and urine specific gravity

Questions

1. Discuss the pathophysiology of multiple myeloma.

2. Discuss clinical manifestations of multiple myeloma.

3. Discuss assessment and diagnostic findings.

4. Discuss different steps of diagnostic staging used to guide and manage treatment of multiple myeloma.

5. Discuss nursing diagnoses for multiple myeloma.

6. Discuss common complications of multiple myeloma.

7. What are the purposes for the prescribed orders?

8. What are the most common adverse reactions to the prescribed medications?

9. Discuss the drug-to-drug and drug-to-food/herbal interactions for the prescribed medications.

10. Discuss client educational for the client with multiple myeloma.

Chronic Myelogenous Leukemia

GENDER

M

AGE

60

SETTING

- Hospital health clinic

ETHNICITY/CULTURE

- White/Portuguese

PREEXISTING CONDITIONS

COEXISTING CONDITIONS

LIFESTYLE

- Retired plastic factory employee

COMMUNICATION

DISABILITY

- Yes

SOCIOECONOMIC STATUS

- Middle

SPIRITUAL/RELIGIOUS

- Anglican

PHARMACOLOGIC

- Imatinib mesylate (Gleevec)
- Leucovorin calcium (Folinic acid)
- Hydroxyurea (Hydrea)
- Interferon alfa-2b (Intron-A)

PSYCHOSOCIAL

- Depression

LEGAL

- If work-related factors are the cause of CML, employers should help with treatment costs, and the client should receive lifelong compensation.

ETHICAL

- Clients should be informed of risk factors in the workplace and educated on how to prevent direct exposure to those risks.

ALTERNATIVE THERAPY

- Naturopathy
- Ginseng
- Soy foods

PRIORITIZATION

- Private room
- Monitor platelet function

DELEGATION

- RN
- Client education

MODERATE

THE CARDIOVASCULAR AND LYMPHATIC SYSTEMS

Level of difficulty: Moderate

Overview: This case involves a thorough history that should include questions pertaining to risk factors and causative factors, occupation, and hobbies to detect causative environmental factors that may have aggravated leukemic process. The case involves questioning the client about frequency and severity of infectious process during the preceding six months, because the risk for infection is increased in clients with leukemia. It requires asking about overt or hidden excessive bleeding episodes, because platelet function is usually diminished with leukemia. Aggressive treatment is needed with chronic myelogenous leukemia (CML), because it can and often does progress to acute leukemia.

Client Profile

Mr. K is a 60-year-old client who came to the hospital outpatient clinic complaining of increased sensitivity at his right side, unusual loss of appetite, and weight loss, which he believes is due to lack of appetite. He reports discomfort in the right and left upper quadrants and informs the nurse that he is concerned about his health because of a family history of leukemia. Mr. K is 5′6″ and weighs 285 pounds. On initial discussion with a nurse, he remarks that he is wondering if his symptoms are early signs of recurring leukemia because he was diagnosed with "childhood leukemia" at the age of 12. However, "he had complete remission" after several treatments at a children's hospital in Portugal. Mr. K reports that he was employed for ten years in a factory that manufactures plastic covers for furniture and household items.

Case Study

Mr. K is known to the clinic and is a reliable historian. Mr. K informs the nurse he has been seeing a naturopathic practitioner, he is currently taking ginseng, and he has recently included soy foods in his diet. The nurse assesses Mr. K and, on physical exam, finds an enlarged spleen and liver and a palpable mass on palpation. Upon completion of the nursing history and assessment, the nurse informs the nurse practitioner (NP) of the findings. The NP continues with further physical assessment on Mr. K and elicits that he has been experiencing weakness, early satiety, and sweating more frequently over the past week. He also reports easy fatigability with minimal activities of daily living (ADLs) and occasional "gouty attacks." After the NP reviews the assessment findings with a medical doctor and a hematologist, the following serum labs are ordered: complete blood count (CBC) with peripheral blood smear, serum acid levels, and alkaline phosphatase. The CBC reveals:

High numbers of mature white blood cells (WBCs): 30,000/mm^3

Decreased hematocrit (Hct): 33.2%

Hemoglobin (Hgb): 12.9%

Platelet counts: elevated at 480,000/mm^3

The peripheral smear reflects the presence of granulocytes at all levels of maturation, serum uric acid level is elevated (9.2 mg/dl), and alkaline phosphatase (LAP score) is reduced (28 U/L). The multidisciplinary team reviews the recent serum lab data and determines that a bone marrow aspiration and biopsy would enhance the diagnosis. Mr. K is informed of the need for the procedures, agrees, and signs an informed witnessed consent. Mr. K is given two oxycodone/acetaminophen 5/325 mg tablets prior to the bone marrow aspiration and biopsy procedure. The bone marrow aspiration and biopsy reveal hypercellularity, megakaryocytosis, and B-cell proliferation. After reviewing the results and report from the hematologist, the oncologist assigns the diagnosis of CML. The health care provider discusses the diagnosis and chemotherapy treatment plan with Mr. K, and refers him to the dietitian, who, in collaboration with the health care team, plans a balanced diet with supplemental vitamins and iron.

The following are prescribed:
- Imatinib mesylate (Gleevec) 400 mg PO four times per day
- Leucovorin calcium (Folinic acid) 10 mg/M^2 IV q6h until serum methotrexate level is less than 0.05 micromolar
- Hydroxyurea (Hydrea) 30 mg/kg PO daily
- Interferon alfa-2b (Intron-A) 2 million U/m^2 three times per week

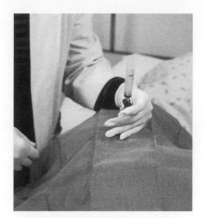

Bone marrow biopsy/aspiration.

Questions

1. Discuss the incidence and prevalence of CML.

2. Discuss the pathophysiology of CML.

3. Discuss diagnostic studies for CML.

4. Discuss main prognostic indicators of CML.

5. Discuss common nursing diagnoses and expected outcome criteria for adult clients with CML.

6. What are the purposes for the prescribed medications?

7. What are the most common adverse reactions of the prescribed medications?

8. Discuss the drug-to-drug and drug-to-food/herbal interactions for the prescribed medications.

9. Discuss health care resources that are usually needed by clients with CML.

10. Discuss client education for CML.

Femoral-Popliteal Bypass for Peripheral Vascular Disease

GENDER

M

AGE

72

SETTING

ETHNICITY/CULTURE

■ White/American

PREEXISTING CONDITIONS

COEXISTING CONDITIONS

LIFESTYLE

■ Retired computer sales manager

COMMUNICATION

DISABILITY

SOCIOECONOMIC STATUS

■ Middle

SPIRITUAL/RELIGIOUS

■ Catholic

PHARMACOLOGIC

■ Morphine sulfate (Duramorph)
■ Dipyridamole (Persantine)
■ Piperacillin sodium/tazobactam sodium (Zosyn)

PSYCHOSOCIAL

■ Anxiety

LEGAL

ETHICAL

ALTERNATIVE THERAPY

PRIORITIZATION

■ Assess and manage pain
■ Peripheral vascular assessment
■ Increase tissue perfusion

DELEGATION

■ RN
■ Client education

MODERATE

THE CARDIOVASCULAR AND LYMPHATIC SYSTEMS

Level of difficulty: Moderate

Overview: This case requires critical post-operative care for the client with peripheral vascular disease. The nurse must use critical decision making in pain management and be able to critically assess for signs or symptoms of reocclusion of the graft.

Client Profile

Mr. T is a 72-year-old male admitted to the surgical intensive care unit (SICU) following a femoral-popliteal bypass graft of the right lower extremity for peripheral vascular disease. Mr. T is initially admitted to the emergency department (ED) of the hospital with complaints of severe pain of the extremity even at rest (ischemic rest pain). He reports a long history of cigarette smoking and history of hypertension and coronary artery disease (atheroclesrosis) and denies surgical history in the past. A Doppler study is done; peripheral pulses of the right extremity are faint and are absent on palpation, peripheral pulses of the left lower extremity are weak, and bilateral extremities are cool to touch.

Case Study

During the history and physical in the ED by a health care provider, Mr. T's pain becomes so unbearable even at rest that he is transported to the operating room for emergency surgery. The surgery is completed, and Mr. T is transferred to the SICU. On arrival, Mr. T is alert but drowsy. However, he moves his head and responds to his name when called, and is responsive to tactile stimuli. He has an arterial line in place, intravenous catheter with Ringer's lactate infusing at 125 mL per hour via electronic pump. He is attached to telemetry, with normal sinus rhythm and occasional unifocal premature ventricular contractions (PVCs) noted. He has a face mask with 40% oxygen in place and a Foley catheter in situ with clear, amber-colored urine draining in a urometer. He has an arterial line in situ, and on arrival to the unit, his vital signs are:

> Blood pressure: 140/82
>
> Pulse: 98
>
> Respirations: 18
>
> Temperature: 99.4° F

His leg is wrapped with a light dressing and orders are written to keep the leg flat in bed. His chart reveals post-embolectomy. The receiving nurse completes the assessment, provides initial care to the client, and proceeds to document the data.

The following are prescribed:
- Morphine sulfate (Duramorph) 2 mg IV q1–2h PRN
- Dipyridamole (Persantine) 100 mg PO four times per day
- Piperacillin sodium/tazobactam sodium (Zosyn) 3 g IV q6h
- Serum PTT, aPTT, CBC, and INR daily
- Bed rest with extremity straight

Questions

1. Discuss the factors from Mr. T's past medical history that predispose him to the need for femoral popliteal bypass.

2. Discuss the femoral-popliteal bypass procedure.

3. Discuss a specific diagnostic test to determine that the bypass procedure is needed and how the test is performed

4. Discuss important post-operative assessment findings to which a nurse should give critical attention.

5. Discuss common nursing diagnoses, expected outcomes, and nursing interventions for the client with post-femoral-popliteal bypass.

6. Discuss the potential complications post femoral-popliteal bypass graft.

7. What are the purposes for the prescribed orders?

8. What are the common adverse reactions, drug-to-drug, drug-to-food/herbal interactions of the prescribed drugs?

9. Discuss client education for post-femoral-popliteal bypass.

CASE STUDY 12

Premature Ventricular Contractions

GENDER

M

AGE

72

SETTING

■ Adult home and hospital

ETHNICITY/CULTURE

■ Black American/West Indian

PREEXISTING CONDITIONS

■ Premature ventricular contractions and atrial fibrillation

COEXISTING CONDITIONS

■ Left-sided heart failure

LIFESTYLE

■ Retired farmer

COMMUNICATION

DISABILITY

■ Reduced ability to perform ADL

SOCIOECONOMIC STATUS

■ Low

SPIRITUAL/RELIGIOUS

■ Anglican

PHARMACOLOGIC

■ Atropine sulfate (Atropine)
■ Amiodarone HcL (Cardarone)
■ Lidocaine HcL (Xylocaine)
■ Carvedilol (Coreg)

PSYCHOSOCIAL

■ Anxiety

LEGAL

ETHICAL

■ Availability of place of residence upon discharge

ALTERNATIVE THERAPY

PRIORITIZATION

■ Stabilize heart rate and rhythm

DELEGATION

■ RN
■ Client education

THE CARDIOVASCULAR AND LYMPHATIC SYSTEMS

Level of difficulty: Difficult

Overview: This case involves a thorough assessment of the client's condition with focus on his cardiac status, including the drugs he is presently on and those brought to the hospital. The case involves prioritization in a triage situation and critical thinking to appropriately delegate and transfer the client to the appropriate unit for continued observation.

Client Profile

Mr. J is a 72-year-old male admitted to the emergency department (ED) from an adult home where he has been living for the past two years. Vital signs on admission are:

Blood pressure: 110/74
Pulse: 54
Respirations: 18
Temperature: 98.4° F

Case Study

On admission, Mr. J is alert and oriented to person, date, and current year. He complains of occasional pressure in his chest, and reports feeling tired and dizzy when he keeps his head down for short periods of time. Past medical history (PMH) reveals myocardial infarction five years ago and current left-sided heart failure. The certified nurse's assistant (CNA) who accompanies him to the ED informs the triage nurse that he self medicates with digoxin (Lanoxin), docusate sodium (Colace), and furosemide (Lasix) daily, but the CNA does not know the dosages of the mentioned medications. A chest X-ray is done and reveals pulmonary congestion and a 12-lead EKG shows decrease tissue perfusion, but no signs of new injury to the myocardium. An IV line is inserted and atropine sulfate 0.5 mg IV administered × one, with a noted increase of heart rate of 68. Mr. J is placed on continuous telemetry that reveals unifocal premature ventricular contractions (PVCs) that developed into coupling then trigeminy. Mr. J complains of chest discomfort, the health care provider is informed and reviews the current serum levels:

Serum digoxin: 2.6 ng/dL
Sodium (Na): 135 mEq/L
Potassium (K+): 3 mEq/L
Blood urea nitrogen (BUN): 15 mg/dL
Calcium: 8.5 mg/dL
Magnesium: 2 mg/dL

The drugs brought to the hospital with the client are reviewed and digoxin and furosemide are held. Mr. J is transferred to the coronary care unit (CCU) with a diagnosis of PVCs.

The following are prescribed:

- Dextrose 5% and 0.45% sodium chloride with 20 mEq KcL IV infusion at 100 ml/hr
- Atropine sulfate (Atropine) 0.5 mg IV q1h PRN for a maximum of 2 mg
- Lidocaine HcL (Xylocaine) 50 mg IV bolus at 20 mg/min, repeat in 5 min, then start infusion of 20 mcg/kg/min immediately after first bolus
- Amiodarone HcL (Cardarone) 150 mg IV over 10 mg followed by 360 mg slow infusion over 6 hours followed by 540 mg at 0.5 mg/min over 18 hours
- Place client on continuous telemetry
- Monitor continuous oxygen saturation/pulse oximetry
- Oxygen to maintain oxygen saturation greater than 94%
- Serial arterial blood gas (ABG)
- Carvedilol (Coreg) 3.125 mg two times per day for two weeks
- Serum digoxin levels two times per day until stable
- Monitor serum sodium, potassium, and magnesium levels

Questions

1. Discuss PVCs or complexes.

2. Discuss some risk factors for the development of PVCs.

3. Discuss the effects of atropine sulfate in treating bradycardia and the development of PVCs.

4. Discuss clinical manifestations of PVCs.

5. Discuss the complications that can result from PVCs, especially in Mr. J's case.

6. Discuss common nursing diagnoses for clients with dysrhythmias.

7. Discuss the reasons why Mr. J's digoxin and furosemide are being held.

8. Discuss the reason digoxin immune fab (Ovine) was not prescribed for Mr. J.

9. What are the purposes of the prescribed orders?

10. What are the most common adverse reactions, drug-to-drug, drug-to-food/herbal interactions of the prescribed medications?

11. Discuss the psychosocial impact of being in an intensive care unit (ICU).

12. Discuss client education for a multiple diagnosis of left-sided heart failure and current episodes of PVCs.

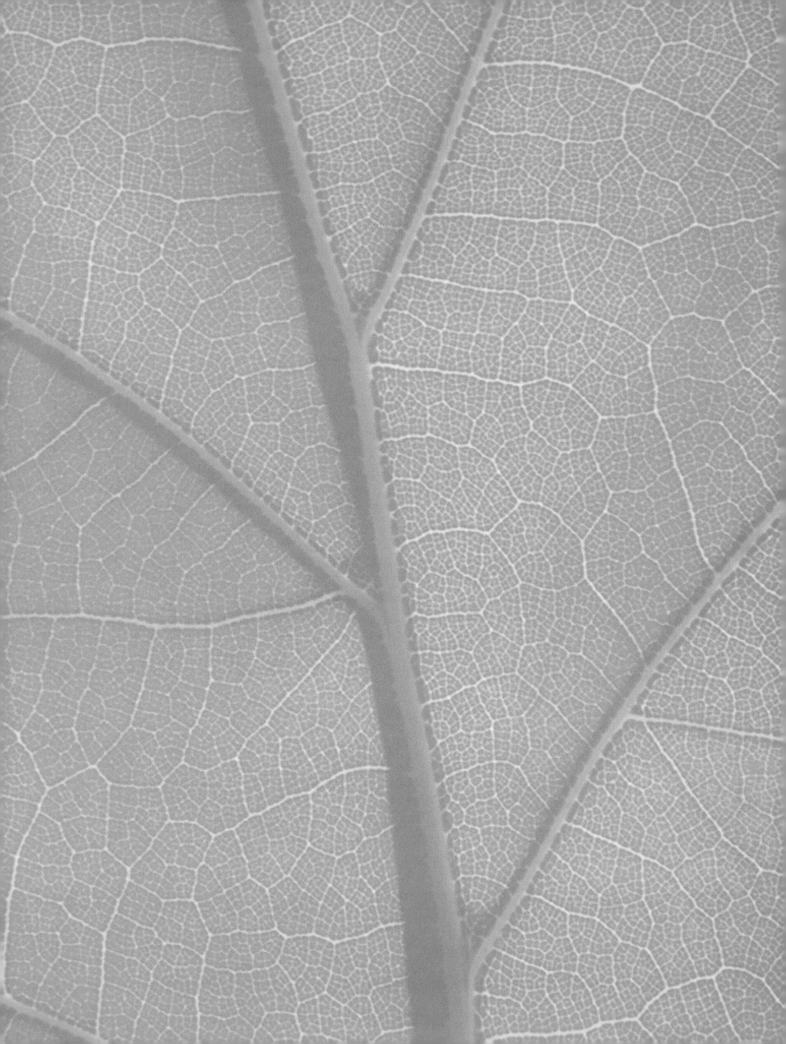

PART FOUR

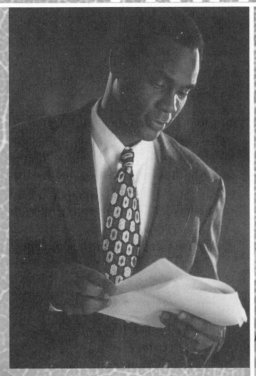

The Nervous System

Unilateral Ménière's Disease

GENDER

M

AGE

30

SETTING

- Clinic

ETHNICITY/CULTURE

- Hispanic American

PREEXISTING CONDITIONS

COEXISTING CONDITIONS

- Allergic reactions to sulfur, feathers

LIFESTYLE

- Licensed mechanic

COMMUNICATION

Spanish and English

DISABILITY

SOCIOECONOMIC STATUS

- Middle

SPIRITUAL/RELIGIOUS

- Evangelical

PHARMACOLOGIC

- Meclizine HcL (Antivert)
- Diazepam (Valium)
- Hydrochlorothiazide (HydroDIURIL)
- Nicotinic acid (Nicobid)
- Dimenhydrinate (Dramamine)

PSYCHOSOCIAL

- Anxiety
- Fear

LEGAL

ETHICAL

- Drugs that cause drowsiness will prohibit the client from working.

ALTERNATIVE THERAPY

PRIORITIZATION

- Maintain safety

DELEGATION

- RN
- Client education

EASY

THE NERVOUS SYSTEM

Level of difficulty: Easy

Overview: This case involves a thorough assessment of the client's condition including all drugs he may be currently taking. The case also involves a careful history for vertigo, the extent of disability, and implementing of measures to stabilize balance.

Client Profile

Mr. S is a 30-year-old single client who is employed by a major motor vehicle department as a licensed mechanic. Mr. S is seen in the clinic with complaints of imbalance, which he relates to a roaring sound and a feeling of fullness in his left ear for the past two weeks. On further history gathering by the nurse, Mr. S reports that periods of whirling infrequently last for a few minutes, but during the past two days, vertigo has lasted for 30 minutes.

Case Study

On further assessment, Mr. S complains of nausea, vomiting, diaphoresis, and a persistent feeling of imbalance, which occurred while he was on the job the previous day, causing him to request time off to seek medical assistance. History and physical are continued by a nurse practitioner (NP), who documents a normal physical examination, with the exception of evaluation of cranial nerve VIII, indicating impairment of the left ear. An audiogram is done, and reveals a sensorineural hearing loss in the left ear. An electronystagmogram is done and shows reduced vestibular response in the left ear. Physical examination findings and diagnostic results are discussed and a diagnosis of Ménière's disease is made in collaboration with a health care provider. Mr. S will be given prescriptions and instructions to return to the clinic in two weeks for follow-up evaluation. The registered dietitian discusses the need for a low sodium diet with Mr. S, and the RN provides him with a list of foods that are both high and low in sodium.

The following are prescribed:
- Meclizine HcL (Antivert) 50 mg PO daily
- Diazepam (Valium) 5 mg PO two times per day
- Hydrochlorothiazide (HydroDIURIL) 50 mg PO daily
- Nicotinic acid (Nicobid) 10 mg PO daily
- Dimenhydrinate (Dramamine) 50 mg PO q6h

Questions

1. Discuss the pathophysiology of Ménière's disease.

2. Discuss the incidence and prevalence of Ménière's disease.

3. Discuss clinical manifestations of Ménière's disease.

4. Discuss diagnostic studies for Ménière's disease.

5. Discuss common nursing diagnoses and goals for vertigo.

6. What are the purposes for the prescribed medications?

7. What are common adverse reactions of the prescribed medications?

8. Discuss drug-to-drug and drug-to-food/herbal interactions of the prescribed medications.

9. Surgical treatment of Ménière's disease is a last resort. When medical therapy is ineffective, discuss surgical procedures that may be performed.

10. Discuss client education for Ménière's disease.

Multiple Sclerosis

GENDER

F

AGE

38

SETTING

- Hospital

ETHNICITY/CULTURE

- White American

PREEXISTING CONDITIONS

COEXISTING CONDITIONS

LIFESTYLE

- Accountant

COMMUNICATION

DISABILITY

- Impaired mobility

SOCIOECONOMIC STATUS

- Middle

SPIRITUAL/RELIGIOUS

- Baptist

PHARMACOLOGIC

- Interferon beta-1a (Avonex)
- Mitoxantrone HcL (Novantrone)
- Baclofen (Lioresal)
- Carbamazepine (Tegretol)
- Methylprednisolone (Medrol)
- Amantadine HcL (Symmetrel)

PSYCHOSOCIAL

- Anxiety
- Emotional instability
- Depression

LEGAL

ETHICAL

- Confidentiality
- Client and family involvement in decision making
- Disability issues
- Quality of life

ALTERNATIVE THERAPY

- Meditation

PRIORITIZATION

- Systems assessment
- Monitor temperature and serum calcium levels

DELEGATION

- RN
- Client education

MODERATE

THE NERVOUS SYSTEM

Level of difficulty: Moderate

Overview: This case uses systems assessment to detect features of multiple sclerosis (MS). It involves a thorough assessment of the client's condition including prescribed drugs and alternative therapy used to help relieve distressing symptoms. The nurse must use critical-thinking skills to prioritize and implement quality care, with the use of therapeutic management aimed at treating the disease process and providing symptomatic relief.

Client Profile

Mrs. N is a 38-year-old married woman with three children, ages 9, 11, and 13. She has been active with her family and community activities. She has worked as a certified accountant in a law firm for more than ten years. Her husband has been employed at a major bank in the city for 15 years. Mrs. N's husband accompanies her to the hospital's emergency department (ED) because of complaints of increased fatigue and stiffness in the lower extremities and double vision. She is 5'8" and weighs 195 pounds. She is a good historian who responds to questions in a detailed manner. Mrs. N denies family history of neurological diseases and reports that her parents are alive and well.

Case Study

Ms. N's complaints on arrival to the ED include increased fatigue and stiffness of the lower extremities with unsteady gait and sudden fuzziness of the eyes followed by double vision (diplopia). She reports that similar symptoms were noticed two years ago, with brief periods of decreased visual acuity that disappeared after a while. Therefore, medical attention was not sought. Mrs. N is transferred to a medical unit of the hospital for continued assessment and evaluation. Her vital signs are:

> Blood pressure: 130/78
>
> Pulse: 78
>
> Respirations: 16
>
> Temperature: 98.6° F

The health care provider completes a thorough history and physical with focus on basic motor skills and sensory assessments which elicited positive indications for MS. A magnetic resonance imaging (MRI) is scheduled and the health care provider discusses ongoing plans with the primary nurse who continues with the nursing history and assessment. Further neurological assessment finds increased deep tendon reflexes, and the client's report of numbness, paresthesia, tingling, and burning in the lower extremities. Babinski reflex is positive, and abdominal reflexes are slow. Serum calcium level is drawn and sent to the lab, revealing a result of 9 mg/dL. The health care provider returns soon after the completion of the nursing assessment with a multidisciplinary team of a neurologist, medical doctor, pharmacist, a nurse practitioner, dietitian, and social worker. After further discussion with Mrs. N pertaining to the physical assessments, the following diagnostic studies are prescribed: Cerebrospinal fluid (CSF) analysis, CSF electrophoresis, MRI of the spine. The neurologist explains the need for a lumbar puncture to Mrs. N and how the procedure would be done. Mrs. N then signs an informed witnessed consent for the lumbar puncture. The social worker remains in the client's room after the rest of the team leaves to discuss the possible need for help at home while she remains in the hospital for continued evaluation. The diagnostic studies are completed and reviewed by the team, then discussed with Mrs. N and her husband as per her request. A diagnosis of MS is confirmed.

The following are prescribed:
- Inteferon beta-1a (Avonex) 30 mcg IM every week
- Mitoxantrone HcL (Novantrone) IV 12 mg/M^2 over 5–15 minutes
- Baclofen (Lioresal) 5 mg PO three times per day
- Methylprednisolone (Medrol) 40 mg PO daily
- Amantadine HcL (Symmetrel) 100 mg PO q12h5

Questions

1. Why is a lumbar puncture used as a diagnostic test for MS?

2. Discuss the guideline for lumbar puncture.

3. What are the expected findings of the diagnostic tests that aided in the confirmation of the diagnosis of MS?

4. What are some common nursing diagnoses for clients with MS?

5. What are the purposes for the prescribed medications?

6. What are the most common adverse reactions of the prescribed medications?

7. Discuss the drug-to-drug and drug-to-food/herbal interactions of the prescribed medications.

8. What are some complementary and alternative therapies that may be included in the comprehensive treatment plan for the client with MS after the client has discussed his or her plan to include these therapies?

9. Why is it important to discharge the client with MS to a rehabilitation center for a brief period of time after discharge from the hospital?

10. Explain a significant psychosocial problem for Mrs. N as it relates to discharge to a rehabilitation center briefly instead of to home.

11. What should the client with MS do to help maintain a sense of well-being upon discharge to home?

Generalized Tonic-Clonic Seizure

GENDER

F

AGE

24

SETTING

- Emergency department

ETHNICITY/CULTURE

- Black American/West Indian

PREEXISTING CONDITIONS

- Head injury two years ago

COEXISTING CONDITIONS

LIFESTYLE

- Nursing student

COMMUNICATION

DISABILITY

SOCIOECONOMIC STATUS

- Middle

SPIRITUAL/RELIGIOUS

- Baptist

PHARMACOLOGIC

- Phenytoin (Dilantin)
- Carbamazepine (Tegretol)
- Diazepam (Valium)

PSYCHOSOCIAL

- Anxiety

LEGAL

- If client injures a person while operating a moving vehicle due to a seizure attack, should the client be liable?

ETHICAL

- Does the client with history of seizure have the right to operate a moving vehicle?

ALTERNATIVE THERAPY

PRIORITIZATION

- Maintain safety
- Control seizure

DELEGATION

- RN
- Client education

THE NERVOUS SYSTEM

Level of difficulty: Difficult

Overview: This case involves a through assessment of the client's presenting symptoms and maintaining a patent airway. The case involves prioritization in a triage situation at a busy urban hospital emergency department (ED).

DIFFICULT

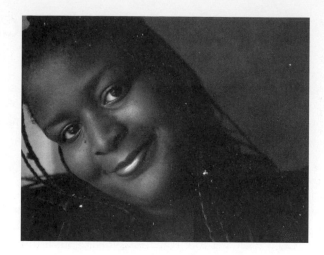

Client Profile

Ms. D is a 24-year-old nursing student who, after leaving the clinic for home via public transportation, complains to her classmates of an unusual feeling that she is not able to describe. A few minutes after her remarks, Ms. D starts to fall but is assisted to the ground by one of her classmates. Emergency medical service (EMS) is contacted, and Ms D's airway is maintained with the help of a passerby while waiting for EMS arrival. The EMS arrives in five minutes and, after a "quick assessment," applies a high-flow oxygen via a non-rebreather mask.

Case Study

Ms. D is taken to the emergency department (ED) of a hospital in a busy section of a large city. On arrival to the hospital triage area, the client is responsive to tactile and verbal stimuli, but not capable of giving an appropriate report of the occurrence. The report is given by a classmate, who describes a tonic phase seizure, with the client uttering a cry then slumping to the ground. The classmate describes Ms. D saying that she felt uneasy and saw unusually bright light, and a smell as though rubber was burning. There was an abrupt increase in muscle tone, loss of consciousness, and loss of postural control, and Ms. D began to fall to the ground but was assisted by her classmate and a passerby. The passerby dialed "911" as the classmate remained with Ms. D. Ongoing observation of Ms. D finds an opisthotonic posture (evidence of acute arching of the back, the head bent back on the neck, the heels bent back on the legs, and the arms and hands flexed rigidly at the joints due to prolonged and severe spasm of the muscles). Ms. D became unconscious, with urinary incontinence; pupils were fixed and dilated, lasting for approximately 45 seconds. Continued observation by the classmate describes alternating contraction and relaxation of the muscles in all the extremities along with hyperventilation. Ms. D is now in the ED, alert, and oriented to her name and place, but not to time of day. A triage nurse continues collection of additional data from the client and her classmate, while an ED clerk notifies the health care provider of Ms. D's arrival. She is placed in a single room, in a side-lying position, and a suction machine and apparatus are at the bedside. Vital signs are:

Blood pressure: 130/80

Pulse: 82

Respirations: 20

Temperature: 98.6° F

Serum labs are drawn: glucose, sodium, total calcium. The bed is placed in low position and side-rails are padded. A stat dose of diazepam (Valium) 10 mg IV is administered by the triage nurse while awaiting the arrival of the health care provider. Thirty minutes after the valium is administered, Ms. D responds appropriately to verbal and tactile stimuli. The health care provider arrives and orders a loading dose of phenytoin which is initiated by the triage nurse. The health care provider continues with a history and physical, history of seizures, psychosocial assessment and mental status examination, and a detailed neurologic examination. Ms. D denies history of seizure or prior episode before today. Upon completion of a neurological assessment, the health care provider orders an electroencephalogram (EEG), and a computed tomography (CT) scan. Result of an ECG shows brain wave abnormalities and the CT scan negative for congenital abnormalities or masses. Based on the documentation of the presenting symptoms on arrival to the ED, and the ECG brain wave abnormalities, a diagnosis of tonic-clonic seizure is confirmed.

The following are prescribed:

- Phenytoin (Dilantin) 100 mg three times per day × seven days then return to health care provider for evaluation
- Carbamazepine (Tegretol) 200 mg PO two times per day
- Complete blood count and serum electrolyte levels
- Carbamazepine and phenytoin levels in the morning

Questions

1. What is the incidence and prevalence of seizure (epilepsy) in the United States?

2. Discuss the pathophysiology of seizures.

3. What is a tonic-clonic seizure?

4. What are common nursing diagnoses for the client with seizure?

5. What is the focus of documentation for a client having a seizure?

6. What is included in the diagnostic assessment of seizures?

7. What are the purposes for the prescribed orders, including diazepam administered in the ED?

8. What are the most common adverse reactions of the prescribed medications, including diazepam?

9. Discuss the drug-to-drug and drug-to-food/herbal interactions for the prescribed medications, including diazepam.

10. What is a major complication of seizure activity?

11. Discuss client education for seizures.

CASE STUDY 4

Subarachnoid Hemorrhage – Grade II

GENDER

F

AGE

42

SETTING

- Hospital

ETHNICITY/CULTURE

- Mixed race

PREEXISTING CONDITIONS

- Hypertension

COEXISTING CONDITIONS

LIFESTYLE

- Bank supervisor

COMMUNICATION

DISABILITY

SOCIOECONOMIC STATUS

- Middle

SPIRITUAL/RELIGIOUS

- Baptist

PHARMACOLOGIC

- Mannitol (Osmitrol)
- Nimodipine (Nimotop)
- Phenobarbital sodium (Luminal Sodium)
- Phenytoin (Dilantin)
- Valsartan (Diovan)
- Ducosate sodium (Colace)

PSYCHOSOCIAL

- Anxiety
- Denial

LEGAL

ETHICAL

ALTERNATIVE THERAPY

PRIORITIZATION

- Brief mental status exam
- Prevent increase in intracranial pressure

DELEGATION

- RN
- Client education

THE NERVOUS SYSTEM

Level of difficulty: Difficult

Overview: This case involves emergency management. The nurse must use critical-thinking skills to prioritize care in a busy triage area to prevent increase in intracranial pressure. The nurse must be skilled and competent at implementing care to maintain cerebral perfusion pressure, controlling intracranial pressure (ICP), managing cardiac dysrhythmias, and preventing rebleeding with ongoing neurologic assessment.

Client Profile

Mrs. M-W is a 43-year-old client who has been experiencing bouts of headache for the past two months. The headaches have become worse, increasing in severity and frequency over the past two weeks. Today, Mrs. M-W experienced a sudden onset of severe headache while preparing a meal for her family. She yells to her husband saying, "I just had a sudden headache that is so severe, I feel weak. It is the worst one I have had." The husband enters the kitchen to find Mrs. M-W projectile vomiting. Mr. W calls his brother-in-law (his neighbor) and they accompany Mrs. M-W to the emergency department (ED) in their community.

Case Study

On arrival at the ED, Mrs. M-W describes the pain as "awful" and sudden. She complains of nausea, and tells the nurse her eyes are blurred. The nurse examines the client, while the certified nursing technician requests that the ED health care provider be paged, then notifies the intensive care unit of the pending transfer. Mrs. M-W is awake, alert, and oriented to person, place, and time. Her conversation and response to questions are comprehensible and easily understood. Mrs. M-W reports a history of hypertension for ten years, and social drinking at dinner time. She is currently taking Valsartan 80 mg PO daily. She follows complex commands, her facial structure is normal, and she is able to move all extremities with equal strength. Her pupils are equal and reactive to light and accommodation. However, her neck is stiff and painful with positive Kernig's and Brudzinski's sign. Her vital signs are:

Blood pressure: 170/96

Pulse: 90

Respirations: 18

Temperature: 98.6° F

The health care provider orders a noncontrast computed tomography (CT) scan of the brain, which reveals blood in the subarachnoid space, intracerebral clots, and large clots surrounding an aneurysm. A transcranial doppler ultrasonography (TCD) is done with evidence of minimal vasospasms. The client is transferred to the medical intensive care unit (MICU) and is placed on complete bed rest, with the head of the bed elevated at 45 degrees, while the nursing team prepares her for possible surgery. An arterial line is inserted, and neurological assessment is ongoing, including blood pressure readings and monitoring of arterial pressure. An intravenous line of D 5.45% NS at 100 mL per hour is initiated. The client is instructed to avoid coughing, sneezing, or straining and is given reasons for these instructions. Bilateral pneumatic compression devices to lower extremities are applied as per protocol for subarachnoid hemorrhage (SAH). Seizure precautions are initiated as per protocol for SAH. After the interdisciplinary team reviews the history and physical and diagnostic studies, the neurologist decides that the diagnosis is grade II SAH secondary to cerebral aneurysm rupture. The treatment plan for a craniotomy is discussed with Mrs. M-W and her husband. An informed consent is signed by Mrs. M-W.

The following are prescribed:
- Neurologic assessment and blood pressure q1h and PRN
- Mannitol (Osmitrol) IV 0.5–1 g/kg over five to ten minutes, may repeat 0.25–1 g/kg q4h per critical-care protocol
- Furosemide (Lasix) 40 mg IV prior to administration of mannitol

- Phenobarbital sodium (Luminal Sodium) 100 mg IV two times per day
- Phenytoin (Dilantin) 1 g loading dose IV, 100 mg q8h
- Nimodipine (Nimotop) 60 mg PO q4h for 21 days. Start in morning
- Ducosate sodium (Colace) 100 mg PO three times per day
- Serum labs: sodium, platelet count
- Insert indwelling urinary catheter
- Hourly urine outputs

Questions

1. Which factors in the case study indicate that Mrs. M-W has suffered an SAH?

2. Discuss precautions to avoid SAH.

3. Discuss the incidence and socioeconomic impact of intracranial aneurysm and SAH.

4. Discuss common nursing diagnoses and expected outcomes for the client with SAH

5. Discuss the conditions that occur after an aneurysm ruptures.

6. Discuss specific factors related to the treatment of SAH that may cause hyponatremia and complications in clients with SAH.

7. Discuss the advantages and disadvantages of early or delayed surgery for SAH.

8. Discuss the types of surgeries that can be done for the client with SAH secondary to ruptured aneurysm.

9. What are the purposes for the prescribed medications?

10. Discuss the most common adverse reactions of the prescribed medications.

11. Discuss drug-to-drug and drug-to-food/herbal interactions for the prescribed medications.

12. Discuss discharge instructions for the client with post-craniotomy related to SAH secondary to cerebral aneurysm.

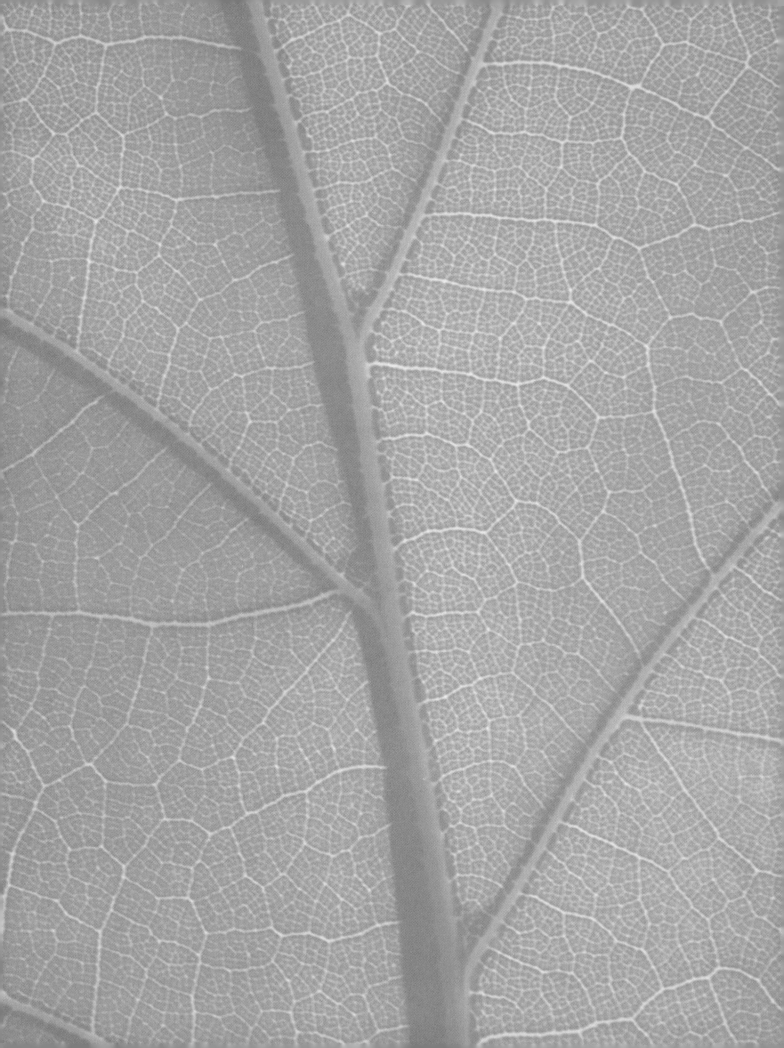

PART FIVE

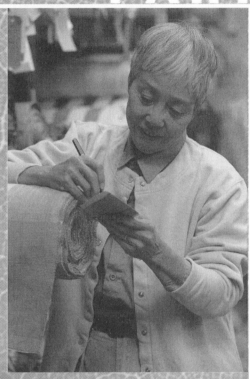

The Endocrine System

Hyperthyroidism

GENDER

F

AGE

30

SETTING

- Family health care provider's office

ETHNICITY/CULTURE

- Black American/West Indian descent

PREEXISTING CONDITIONS

COEXISTING CONDITIONS

LIFESTYLE

- Telephone installer, graduate student

COMMUNICATION

- English

DISABILITY

SOCIOECONOMIC STATUS

- Middle

SPIRITUAL/RELIGIOUS

- Believes in God

PHARMACOLOGIC

- Propylthiouracil (PTU)
- Propranolol HcL (Inderal)

PSYCHOSOCIAL

- Anxiety

LEGAL

ETHICAL

ALTERNATIVE THERAPY

PRIORITIZATION

- Avoid post-operative complication (thyroid storm)
- Maintain cardiac reserve

DELEGATION

- RN
- Client education

THE ENDOCRINE SYSTEM

Level of difficulty: Easy

Overview: This case involves thorough assessment of the client's condition including health history. Physical assessment should focus on testing muscle strength, vital signs, size of thyroid, and presence of bruits over the thyroid gland. The nurse must use critical thinking to prioritize care in a busy triage area in the event the client goes into thyroid crisis.

Client Profile

Ms. C is a 30-year-old female who is employed as a telephone installer for a major cable company. She is 5′7″ with previous weight of 200 pounds. She is presently pursuing a masters degree in telecommunication. Ms. C lives with her parents, but reports that she pays rent for a one-bedroom apartment in her parent's home.

Case Study

Ms. C is seen at her family health care provider's office for follow-up review of observed patterns of behavior and changes in health status over the past month. On interview by the nurse, Ms. C reports unusual hunger, even after having a large meal. She has noted unusual weight loss that is not related to exercise or stress, diarrhea, and inability to tolerate normal heat that she would have not responded to in the past. On assessment, her vital signs are:

Blood pressure: 150/92

Pulse: 120

Respirations: 22

Temperature 101.6° F

She has visible tremors of the hands and her eyeballs are beginning to protrude. Current diagnostic studies reveal abnormal T_3, T_4, and TSH results.

Serum calcium level: 11.2 mg/dL

Red blood cell (RBC) count: 7/mm^3

White blood cell (WBC) count: 4,000/mm^3

Platelet count (PLT): 250,000 /mm^3

Hematocrit (Hct): 34%

Hemoglobin (Hgb): 14 g/100 mL

A thyroid scan with the use of radioactive tracers reveals an enlarged thyroid goiter with increased iodine uptake. Ms. C denies difficulty swallowing or pain upon swallowing. A diagnosis of hyperthyroidism is made by the health care provider, and is discussed with Ms. C, and the possibility for surgery is explained.

The following are prescribed:

- Weekly monitoring of WBC after initiation of PTU
- Propylthiouracil (PTU) 450 mg PO daily
- Strong iodine solution 4 drops three times per day × ten days
- Propranolol HcL (Inderal) 80 mg PO q6h

Questions

1. Discuss the risk factors and pathophysiology of hyperthyroidism.

2. Discuss clinical manifestations of hyperthyroidism.

3. Discuss diagnostic findings of hyperthyroidism.

4. Discuss gerontologic considerations of hyperthyroidism.

5. What are the purposes for the prescribed orders?

6. What are the most common adverse reactions, drug-to-drug, drug-to-food/herbal interactions for the prescribed medications?

7. Discuss complications of hyperthyroidism.

8. Discuss surgical management for hyperthyroidism.

9. Discuss relapse rate and risk for hyperthyroidism after treatment for thyroid storm.

10. Discuss client education for hyperthyroidism.

CASE STUDY 2

Hypercortisolism (Cushing's Syndrome)

GENDER

F

AGE

42

SETTING

- Hospital

ETHNICITY/CULTURE

- Native American/Argentina

PREEXISTING CONDITIONS

- Hypertension

COEXISTING CONDITIONS

- History of alcohol abuse

LIFESTYLE

- Self employed, Indian art antique shop

COMMUNICATION

- Spanish and English

DISABILITY

SOCIOECONOMIC STATUS

- Middle

SPIRITUAL/RELIGIOUS

- Roman Catholic

PHARMACOLOGIC

- Mitotane (Lysodren)

PSYCHOSOCIAL

- Emotional instability
- Irritability
- Depression

LEGAL

- Does the client have the right to bring charges against health care providers if necessary treatment is withheld?

ETHICAL

- Will the client have equitable access to essential health care benefits compared to clients with major medical health coverage?

ALTERNATIVE THERAPY

- Prayer

PRIORITIZATION

- Decrease cortisol levels
- Decrease blood glucose levels
- Provide safety

DELEGATION

- RN
- Client education

MODERATE

THE ENDOCRINE SYSTEM

Level of difficulty: Moderate

Overview: This case involves a thorough assessment of the client's condition, including questions related to recent onset of weakness, increase in weight or abdominal girth, bone pain or history of fractures, and history of frequent infections and easy bruising. It involves questioning the client about gastrointestinal (GI) discomfort and the use of steroid drugs and herbals. The nurse must use critical-thinking skills to prioritize care in the event of signs and symptoms indicating the development of adrenal crisis.

Client Profile

Mrs. V is a 42-year-old widow whose husband and only child, who was three years old, died in a motor vehicle accident three years ago, the day before Christmas. Prior to their deaths, Mrs. V and her husband of 12 years had wine as a social appetizer during meal times. Mrs. V is 5′4″ and weighs 208 pounds.

Case Study

Mrs. V reports that since her husband's death, she has continued with the practice of having wine with her evening meals. However, she reports that as the years went by, she became lonely, missing her husband and child, especially at holidays, which led to an increase in the amount of wine consumed at meal times. The client reports social drinking with her friends who frequently visit her at the "shop" at which she worked as manager. The client's husband was a real estate broker for a progressive brokerage firm. Mrs. V finds out she had no health insurance when she goes to a community health center for elevated blood pressure and ongoing headaches. Her blood pressure at the time of arrival was 194/98 and she complained of nausea. A history is taken by a nurse practitioner (NP) at the clinic and Mrs. V is referred to the community hospital emergency department (ED), and transported from the clinic to the community hospital. On arrival at the ED, she informs the triage nurse that the headache is less severe in comparison to when she was at the clinic. Mrs. V believes the headache is directly related to her history of hypertension. The NP does the history and physical in the ED, during which time Mrs. V reports periods of emotional instability, with mood swings and depression. She informs the nurse that at times she is unusually irritable for no specific reasons, and experiences frequent urination, muscle weakness, and easy bruising. Physical assessment findings reveal hirsutism and a male pattern type balding of the head, abdominal striae, and dependent edema of the lower extremities. Mrs. V is admitted to a medical unit and will be seen by an endocrinologist for further evaluation. The primary nurse assigned to Mrs. V completes additional nursing history and assessment, after which Mrs. V is seen by an endocrinologist. The following tests are ordered: 24-hour urine for free cortisol and 17-hydroxycorticosteroids and 17-ketosteroids, plasma cortisol, ACTH level, erythro-sedimentation rate (ESR), white blood cell (WBC) count, lymphocyte count, sodium, potassium, and calcium, urine calcium, potassium, and glucose. A computed tomography (CT) of the adrenal gland is ordered, and a high-dose (8 mg) dexamethasone suppression test is ordered for the next day. The nurse instructs Mrs. V on how to collect the 24-hour urine and received verbal feedback that was positive. The results of the diagnostic studies reveal 24-hour urine for 17-hydroxycorticosteroids and 17-ketosteroids elevated (12 mg/24 h), and:

Plasma cortisol: 30 ug/dL

ACTH in AM: 100 pg/mL; in PM: 75 pg/mL

Erythro-sedimentation rate (ESR): elevated

White blood cell (WBC) count: 12,000/mm^3

Lymphocyte count: 700/mm^3

Sodium (Na): 150 mEq/L

Decrease potassium (K+): 2.8 mEq/L

Calcium: 7 mg/dL

Increase glucose: 140 mg/dL

Urine calcium: 310 mg/24 h, elevated

Urine potassium: 150 mEq/24 h

Urine glucose: 300 mg/24 h

The high dose dexamethasone suppression test reveals reduction in plasma cortisol level less than 50% of the baseline, indicating positive finding for Cushing's syndrome. The CT scan reveals an inoperable adrenal tumor. An endocrinologist reviews the labs and diagnostic reports with the multidisciplinary team; a diagnosis of Cushing's syndrome is confirmed. The multidisciplinary team discusses the plan of care with Mrs. V, and she agrees with the plan.

The following is prescribed:

- Mitotane (Lysodren) 3 g PO three times per day

Questions

1. Discuss the prevalence and pathophysiology of Cushing's syndrome.

2. Discuss clinical manifestations of Cushing's syndrome.

3. Discuss assessment and diagnostic findings of Cushing's syndrome.

4. Discuss common nursing diagnoses for Cushing's syndrome.

5. Discuss a potential complication of Cushing's syndrome.

6. What is the purpose for the prescribed medication?

7. What are the most common adverse reactions, drug-to-drug, drug-to-food/herbal interactions of the prescribed medications?

8. Discuss adrenalectomy for primary adrenal hypertrophy in Cushing's syndrome.

9. Discuss management of adrenal insufficiency post adrenalectomy.

10. Discuss client education after bilateral adrenalectomy.

CASE STUDY 3

Diabetes Mellitus Type 1

GENDER

M

AGE

20

SETTING

- Hospital

ETHNICITY/CULTURE

- Hispanic American

PREEXISTING CONDITIONS

- Viral infection

COEXISTING CONDITIONS

- Father and grandmother have history of diabetes

LIFESTYLE

- College student
- Basketball team member
- Lives with family

COMMUNICATION

- Spanish and English

DISABILITY

SOCIOECONOMIC STATUS

- Middle

SPIRITUAL/RELIGIOUS

- Evangelical

PHARMACOLOGIC

- Human regular (Novolin-R)
- Sodium bicarbonate
- Insulin aspart (NovoLog)

PSYCHOSOCIAL

- Anxiety
- Depression

LEGAL

ETHICAL

ALTERNATIVE THERAPY

PRIORITIZATION

- Assessment for signs and symptoms of pending complications
- Administering prescribed medications

DELEGATION

- RN
- LPN
- Client education

THE ENDOCRINE SYSTEM

Level of difficulty: Moderate

Overview: This case involves a thorough assessment of the presenting symptoms on arrival to triage, including all medications the client is currently taking. It involves critical thinking to appropriately delegate assignment to nurses highly competent in applying decision-making skills to clients requiring immediate medical and nursing interventions. The nurse must be capable of identifying pending signs of diabetic complications and able to collaborate with the team to prevent occurrences.

Client Profile

Mr. J is a 20-year-old college student with a history of diabetes mellitus type 1 for the past six years. Mr. J lives at home with his extended family. Mr. J's father and grandmother have a history of diabetes mellitus type 1. Mr. J is the only other member of the family diagnosed with the disease.

Case Study

Mr. J is a respiratory therapist major at a community college and is a member of the basketball team. Mr. J is brought to the emergency department (ED) by emergency medical services after Mr. J collapsed during basketball practice at the college. A member of the basketball team accompanies Mr. J in the ambulance. Mr. J is 6'3" and weighs 220 pounds. His family is notified by college authorities and arrives at the ED while Mr. J is being triaged. On arrival at the ED, he is responsive to verbal and tactile stimuli, is very diaphoretic, mildly lethargic, and is complaining of abdominal pain and nausea. He hyperventilates, manifesting acetone breath. Stat serum glucose, arterial blood gas (ABG), and serum electrolytes for sodium and potassium are done and reveal:

> Blood glucose: 450 mg/dL
>
> pH: 6.9
>
> pCO_2: 20 mm Hg
>
> HCO_3: 12 mEq/L
>
> Sodium (Na): 128 mEq/L
>
> Potassium (K+): 3.0 mEq/L

His vital signs on admission are:

> Blood pressure: 100/70
>
> Pulse: 88, rapid but regular
>
> Respirations: 22
>
> Temperature: 98.1° F

Mr. J is seen by the ED health care provider, and a diagnosis of diabetic ketoacidosis (DKA) is made. Mr. J is transferred to the medical intensive care unit (MICU).

The following are prescribed:

- 0.9% NaCL at 1 liter per hour × two hours
- Human regular (Novolin-R) initial bolus 0.4 units/kg, followed by 2.4 u/hr continuous infusion
- Sodium bicarbonate ($NaHCO_3$) 5 mEq/kg infusion over four hours and low dose insulin at a continuous rate (five units per hour) at 25 mL per hour.
- Monitor serum glucose and potassium level; if stable, change infusion to 0.45% sodium chloride at 125 mL/hr
- Insulin aspart (NovoLog) insulin 100 U/mL inj four units and NPH ten units in combination SC three times per day, before meals

Questions

1. What are specific cultural considerations of diabetes mellitus?

2. What is an extremely critical indicator of diabetes mellitus?

3. What are common nursing diagnoses for clients with diabetes?

4. What is a primary collaborative problem for Mr. J because of the elevated blood glucose level on arrival to the ED?

5. What are the defining characteristics of DKA?

6. What are the priorities of management for a client experiencing DKA?

7. What are the purposes for the prescribed orders?

8. What are the most common adverse reactions of the prescribed medications?

9. Discuss the drug-to-drug and drug-to-food/herbal interactions for the prescribed medications.

10. Explain the difference between Dawn phenomenon and Somogyi phenomenon.

11. What are the critical areas that should be included in client education for type 1 diabetes mellitus?

12. What are the nursing implications as they relate to diabetes mellitus?

CASE STUDY 4

Addison's Disease (Acute-Primary Hypocortisolism)

MODERATE

GENDER

F

AGE

50

SETTING

- Hospital

ETHNICITY/CULTURE

- White American

PREEXISTING CONDITIONS

- History of pulmonary TB

COEXISTING CONDITIONS

- Pernicious anemia

LIFESTYLE

- Clothing designer

COMMUNICATION

DISABILITY

SOCIOECONOMIC STATUS

- Middle

SPIRITUAL/RELIGIOUS

- Methodist

PHARMACOLOGIC

- Hydrocortisone (Hydrocortone)
- Fludrocortisone acetate (Florinef)

PSYCHOSOCIAL

- Depression

LEGAL

ETHICAL

ALTERNATIVE THERAPY

- Vegetarian

PRIORITIZATION

- Prevent Addisonian Crisis
- Maintain safety

DELEGATION

- RN
- Client education

THE ENDOCRINE SYSTEM

Level of difficulty: Moderate

Overview: This case involves a thorough assessment of the client's condition, including current medications and dietary regimen. It involves prioritization in a triage situation at a busy hospital emergency department (ED) to avoid Ms. X developing Addisonian Crisis.

147

Client Profile

Ms. X is a 50-year-old client who is seen in a hospital's outpatient clinic as follow-up to her primary health care provider's referral for diagnostic tests to rule out diagnosis of Addison's disease. During an interview by a registered nurse (RN), she reveals past history of pulmonary tuberculosis and fungal lesions of the skin. She reports currently taking oral vitamin B_{12} for history of pernicious anemia. On further collection of data, Ms. X reports weakness, fatigue, anorexia, nausea, vomiting, and weight loss during the past month. Ms. X visited her primary health care provider a month ago because of dizziness and weakness, when rising from bed in the mornings or when standing from a sitting position for an extended period of time. Initial vital signs on arrival to the clinic are:

Blood pressure: 90/64

Pulse: 126

Respirations: 14

Temperature: 98.9° F

Case Study

Physical assessment of Ms. X reveals hyperpigmentation of the hands and lower extremities. Ms. X is later seen by a physician assistant (PA) who completes the history and physical, and informs Ms. X she will be admitted to the hospital for short-term stay. Serum cortisol, fasting blood glucose, sodium, potassium, blood urea nitrogen (BUN), adrenocortical thyroid hormone (ACTH), and eosinophil count are sent to the lab. The results are:

Serum cortisol: 12 ug/dL

Fasting blood glucose: 50 mg/100 mL

Sodium (Na): 128 mEq/L

Potassium (K+): 6 mEq/dL

Blood urea nitrogen (BUN): 26 mg/100 mL

The ACTH stimulation test reveals 100 pg/mL at 6 to 8 AM (after the patient followed a low-carbohydrate diet for 48 hours and fasted from foods for 12 hours before the test). A computed tomography (CT) with contrast reveals beginning atrophy of the adrenal gland, and magnetic resonance imaging (MRI) is negative for tumors or infections. Urinary 17-hydroxycorticosteroids and 17-ketosteroid levels urinary free cortisol are explained to Ms. X and the procedures are appropriately completed. The result reveals low normal levels. After laboratory data and diagnostic tests are reviewed by an endocrinologist and a medical and nursing staff, the diagnosis of Addison's disease is confirmed. The findings, confirmation of the disease, and treatment plan are discussed with Ms. X.

The following are prescribed:

- Hydrocortisone (Hydrocortone) 30 mg IV three times per day
- Fludrocortisone acetate (Florinef) 0.1 mg PO daily

Questions

1. Discuss the incidence, prevalence, and pathophysiology of Addison's disease.

2. Discuss risk factors of Addison's disease.

3. Discuss clinical manifestations of Addison's disease.

4. Discuss nursing diagnoses for Addison's disease.

5. Discuss diagnostic findings of Addison's disease.

6. Discuss urinary 17-hydroxycorticosteroids.

7. What are the purposes for the prescribed medications?

8. What are the most common adverse reactions, drug-to-drug, drug-to-food/herbal interactions for the prescribed medications?

9. Discuss management of hyponatremia and hyperkalemia found in Addison's disease.

10. Discuss client education for Addison's disease.

CASE STUDY 5

Pheochromocytoma

GENDER

F

AGE

56

SETTING

- Health care provider's office

ETHNICITY/CULTURE

- Black American, West Indian descent

PREEXISTING CONDITIONS

- History of cigarette smoking

COEXISTING CONDITIONS

- Hypertension

LIFESTYLE

- RN

COMMUNICATION

DISABILITY

SOCIOECONOMIC STATUS

- Middle

SPIRITUAL/RELIGIOUS

- Nondenominational

PHARMACOLOGIC

- Furosemide (Lasix)
- Acetaminophen (Tylenol)
- Propranolol HcL (Inderal)
- Prazosin HcL (Minipress)

PSYCHOSOCIAL

- Anxiety

LEGAL

ETHICAL

ALTERNATIVE THERAPY

PRIORITIZATION

- Decrease release of epinephrine and norepinephrine
- Stabilize blood pressure

DELEGATION

- RN
- Client education

THE ENDOCRINE SYSTEM

Level of difficulty: Moderate

Overview: This case involves a thorough assessment of the client's condition, including all current medications she is taking. It involves history and physical examination to gather appropriate data to aid in confirming a diagnosis. The nurse must use critical-thinking skills to prioritize care in the event hypertensive crisis develops.

Client Profile

Ms. P is a 56-year-old female who is seen at her primary health care provider's office after experiencing severe headaches. The nurse at the health care provider's office initiates the initial interview. Ms. P's vital signs are:

Blood pressure: 250/110

Pulse: 114, rapid and regular

Respirations: 20

Temperature: 98.4° F

An electrocardiogram (EKG) is ordered and reveals sinus tachycardia. Ms. P denies other medical problems but admits to years of cigarette smoking, which she stopped 15 years ago. Ms. P reports wearing glasses for distance reading but denies blurred vision. Medication history reveals furosemide (Lasix) 50 mg PO daily, amlodipine (Norvasc) 10 mg PO daily, propranolol HcL (Inderal) 40 mg PO two times per day, and acetaminophen (Tylenol) 650 mg PO PRN headache. She reports occasional constipation and uses increased roughage in the diet, which helps ease defecation. Her parents and siblings are alive and well. Ms. P is referred to the community hospital emergency department (ED) because of the elevated blood pressure.

Case Study

On arrival at the ED, Ms. P's vital signs are:

Blood pressure: 250/100

Pulse: 120, rapid and regular

Respirations: 18

Temperature: 98.4° F

She is transferred to a telemetry unit and is seen by a physician assistant (PA), who completes a history and physical while avoiding vigorous abdominal palpation. Ms. P is transferred to a medical unit and the following order is prescribed: nitroprusside sodium (Nitropress) 0.5 mg/kg per minute stat via infusion pump. Serum lab tests ordered are: sodium (Na), potassium (K+), glucose and urine glucose, 24-hour urine collections for vanillylmandelic acid (VMA), computed tomography (CT) scan of the adrenal gland, and abdominal imaging techniques. The results of the serum labs reveal:

Sodium (Na): 145 mEq/L

Potassium (K+): 4 mEq/L

Glucose: 130 mg/dL

Positive glucosuria

The 24-hour urine collections result reveal slight elevation in metanephrine and catecholamines, the CT scan identifies an adrenomedullary tumor on the left adrenal gland, measuring 0.5 cm, but abdominal imaging techniques are negative for metastasis of the tumor. An endocrinology consult is ordered for a team conference to determine surgical interventions. After the health care provider reviews the current labs and diagnostic findings, a diagnosis of pheochromocytoma is made. The health care team decides to begin treatment of the presenting symptoms while waiting for the endocrinology consult. The treatment plans are discussed with Ms. P Her blood pressure is currently 130/80, and her pulse is 102 and regular. She denies headache at this time. The registered dietitian discusses the dietary plan of care with Ms. P. The endocrinologist reviews the collected data, and determines that Ms. P can be monitored on an outpatient basis, and orders repeat CT scan and abdominal X-rays for three months from today's date. Ms. P will be discharged to home within 24 hours and will have follow-up visits with her primary health care provider.

The following are prescribed:

- Prazosin HcL (Minipress) 1 mg PO daily with gradual increase to 6 mg PO daily
- Propranolol HcL (Inderal) 40 mg PO two times per day
- Furosemide (Lasix) 50 mg PO daily
- Acetaminophen (Tylenol) 650 mg PO PRN headache

Questions

1. Discuss the incidence, prevalence, risk factors, and pathophysiology of pheochromocytoma.

2. Discuss clinical manifestations of pheochromocytoma.

3. Discuss assessment and diagnostic findings of pheochromocytoma.

4. Discuss nursing diagnoses to pheochromocytoma.

5. What are the purposes for the prescribed medications?

6. What are most common adverse reactions, drug-to-drug, drug-to-food/herbal interactions of the prescribed medications?

7. Discuss pre-operative intervention for surgical intervention for pheochromocytoma.

8. Discuss surgical management of pheochromocytoma.

9. Discuss client education for pheochromocytoma.

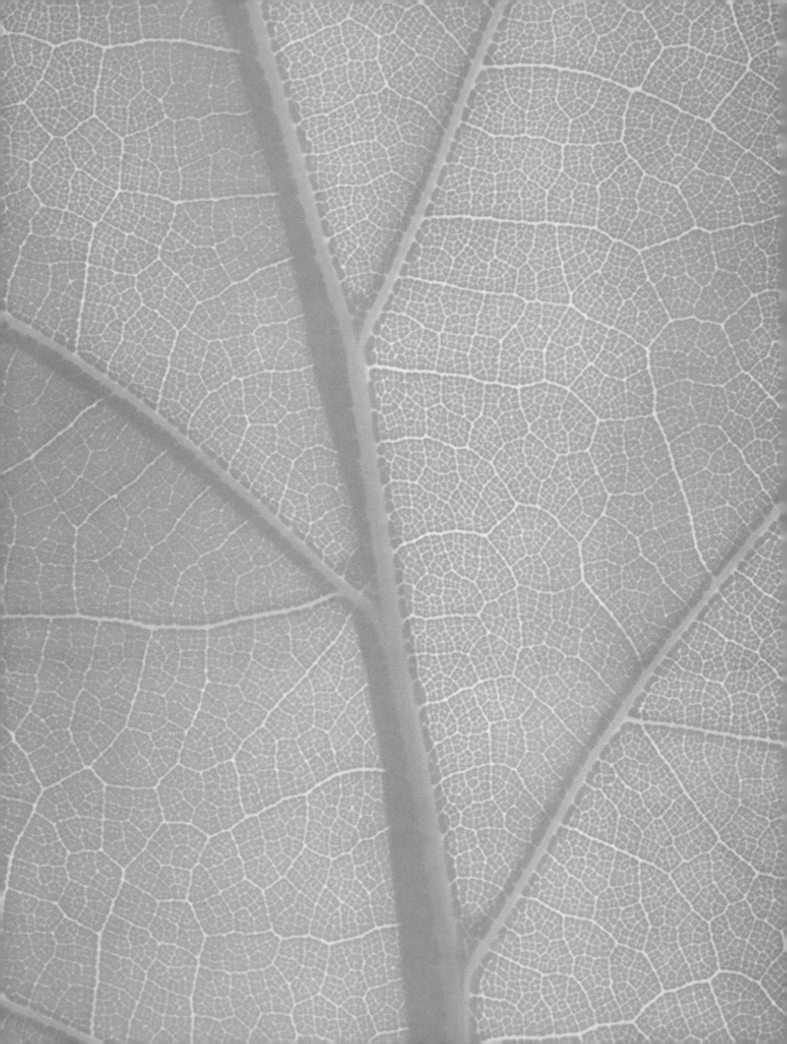

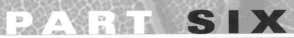

PART SIX

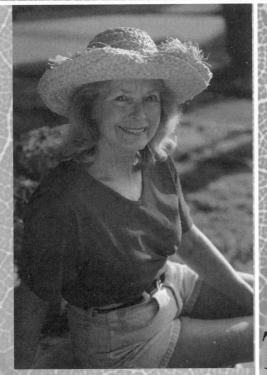

The Musculoskeletal and Reproductive Systems

Cervical Cancer Stage IA

GENDER

F

AGE

25

SETTING

- Women's well clinic of a medical center

ETHNICITY/CULTURE

- Native American

PREEXISTING CONDITIONS

- HPV infection

COEXISTING CONDITIONS

- Squamous intraepithelial lesion

LIFESTYLE

- Unemployed college student
- Lives with sister

COMMUNICATION

DISABILITY

SOCIOECONOMIC STATUS

- Low

SPIRITUAL/RELIGIOUS

- Nondenominational

PHARMACOLOGIC

- Codeine sulfate

PSYCHOSOCIAL

- Anxiety
- Fear

LEGAL

ETHICAL

ALTERNATIVE THERAPY

- Meditation

PRIORITIZATION

- Encourage verbalization of feelings
- Prepare for cryosurgery

DELEGATION

- RN
- Client education

EASY

THE MUSCULOSKELETAL AND REPRODUCTIVE SYSTEMS

Level of difficulty: Easy

Overview: The case involves a thorough and sensitive assessment of the client's condition, taking into account the client's cultural views on health, wellness, and treatment. The nurse must use communication skills that will enhance trust and optimize the nurse–client relationship.

Client Profile

Ms. R is a 25-year-old female college student who is seen in the women's health clinic of a medical center due to complaints of spotting between menstruation. Ms. R is 5'5" and weighs 120 pounds.

Case Study

Ms. R reports to the nurse practitioner (NP) on initial interview that her most recent Papanicolaou test (Pap) test is positive and that she had an appointment to see her family health care provider but missed the scheduled date, and the health care provider is away on personal business with an indefinite time of return. She admits to be being sexually active with the same partner for the past five years. Her reason for coming to the women's clinic is due to "spotting between menstruation" at the time of her last menstrual cycle. However, she is not "spotting" at the time of this visit. Her vital signs on admission are:

Blood pressure: 124/78

Pulse: 78 and regular

Respirations: 18

Temperature: 98.6° F

After continuing the history and physical, the NP discusses the need for further diagnostic evaluation, and when it is ascertained that Ms. R understands the need for the presented evaluation, the NP does a pelvic examination, a colposcopy, and an endocervical curettage. After the procedures, specimens are sent to the lab for analysis. Ms. R's vital signs are repeated and reveal:

Blood pressure: 128/80

Pulse: 80

Respirations: 18

Temperature: 98.6° F

The NP gives Ms. R an appointment for follow-up visit and informs her that at the time of that visit, the results of the colposcopy and endocervical curettage will be discussed with her.

The following are prescribed:

- Contact the clinic if you are experiencing excessive bleeding, discharge, or abdominal pain.

- Return to the clinic in one month for discussion on the results of the specimens sent to the lab.

- Codeine sulfate 15 mg PO q6h PRN

Questions

1. Discuss the etiology and pathophysiology of cervical cancer.

2. Discuss cultural and ethnic considerations of cervical cancer.

3. Discuss clinical manifestations of cervical cancer.

4. Discuss diagnostic studies used to confirm cervical cancer.

5. What is the purpose for the prescribed medication?

6. What are the most common adverse reactions, drug-to-drug, and drug-to-food/herbal interactions of the prescribed medication?

7. Discuss surgical management for cervical cancer.

8. Discuss the clinical stages of cervical cancer.

9. Discuss client education for cervical cancer.

CASE STUDY 2

Closed Femoral Head Fracture
(Intracapsular Fracture)

GENDER

- M

AGE

- 32

SETTING

- Hospital

ETHNICITY/CULTURE

- Black American/West Indian

PREEXISTING CONDITIONS

COEXISTING CONDITIONS

LIFESTYLE

- Professional painter

COMMUNICATION

DISABILITY

SOCIOECONOMIC STATUS

- Middle

SPIRITUAL/RELIGIOUS

- Methodist

PHARMACOLOGIC

- Morphine sulfate (Duramorph)
- Enoxaparin sodium (Lovenox)
- Docusate sodium (Colace)

PSYCHOSOCIAL

- Anxiety
- Pain

LEGAL

- Worker's compensation should be available until client returns to work.

ETHICAL

ALTERNATIVE THERAPY

PRIORITIZATION

- Stabilize extremity
- Assess and manage pain
- Assess neurological status of lower extremities

DELEGATION

- RN
- CNA
- Client education

THE MUSCULOSKELETAL AND REPRODUCTIVE SYSTEMS

Level of difficulty: Easy

Overview: This case first involves assessment of all major body systems for life-threatening complications, including head, thoracic, and abdominal injuries. The case involves assessment of pain and assessment of the skin for intactness, color, temperature, movement, sensation, pulses, and capillary refill. The triage nurse uses critical thinking to appropriately prioritize care of clients with hip dislocation in a busy emergency department (ED). The certified nursing attendant (CNA) can take vital signs and monitor the client for signs of bleeding, such as restlessness, or unusual findings on the skin (e.g., bruising) and inform the nurse.

Client Profile

Mr. P is a 32-year-old painter who is brought to the ED via emergency medical services (EMS) after falling from a ladder while painting a building under contract by his employer. He is 5′9″ and weighs 150 pounds.

Case Study

On arrival to the ED, Mr. P is alert, oriented to time, person and place, but is voicing intolerable pain in the right thigh with slight movement and moderate pain over his entire back. He denies known allergies to foods or drugs or the use of herbals. Vital signs reveal:

> Blood pressure: 130/80
>
> Pulse: 90
>
> Respirations: 20
>
> Temperature: 98.6° F

He is medicated with morphine 10 mg IM for pain as prescribed. Serum labs done in the ED reveal:

> Hematocrit (Hct): 36%
>
> Hemoglobin (Hgb): 14%
>
> Serum calcium: 9 mg/dL
>
> Serum phosphorous: 4 mg/dL

Mr. P is transferred from the stretcher that he is brought in on to a ED bed. His right leg remains immobilized by a long backboard. An EMS personnel provides the triage nurse with a detailed report of physical findings and neurovascular status of the injured extremity on arrival to the injury site. The ED health care provider arrives and after gathering additional pertinent history, the health care provider examines Mr. P for other bony injuries and a careful knee examination is also done. Mr. P is transferred to the orthopedic unit, weighed on a bedscale, then placed on bed rest. A complete assessment is done, including assessment of abrasions and other injuries. An EKG shows normal sinus rhythm, and a chest X-ray is negative for rib fracture or diaphragmatic damage. A venography is negative for pulmonary embolism. A pulse oximeter is initiated with a noted oxygen saturation of 98%. At a later time during the shift, a computed tomography (CT) of the spine, pelvis, hip, and leg is done and reveals an intact spine and pelvis, dislocation of the femoral head, and soft tissue damage of the leg and thigh, but no pre-existing disorders. After the multidisciplinary team reviews the data of diagnostic studies and physical findings, a diagnosis of closed femoral head dislocation is made, and plans for surgery are discussed with Mr. P. He is informed that no food or fluids should be taken (NPO) after a scheduled time in preparation for the surgical procedure. A closed reduction/internal fixation of the femoral head is scheduled. An intravenous (IV) line is initiated with IV solution of 0.9% sodium chloride at 125 mL/hr, and a trapeze is placed over the bed with instructions given to Mr. P on its purpose and use.

The following are prescribed:

- Complete bed rest
- Morphine sulfate (Duramorph) 1–2 mg IV PRN for pain
- Enoxaparin sodium (Lovenox) 100 mg/1mL SC daily
- Docusate sodium (Colace) 100 mg PO three times per day

Questions

1. Discuss the different types of fractures, including the closed fracture.

2. Discuss clinical manifestations of clients with closed femoral head fracture.

3. Discuss the potential complications of a closed femoral head fracture.

4. Discuss the use of crutches instead of a walker for this client.

5. Discuss the teaching guidelines for crutch walking.

6. What are common nursing diagnoses for clients with closed femoral head fracture?

7. What are expected outcomes for clients with closed femoral head fracture?

8. What are the purposes for the prescribed orders?

9. What are the most common adverse reactions, drug-to-drug, drug-to-food/herbal interactions for the prescribed medications?

10. Discuss discharge plans for the client following immobilization of the femoral head fracture.

Osteomyelitis of Left Foot

GENDER

M

AGE

64

SETTING

- Hospital

ETHNICITY/CULTURE

- White American

PREEXISTING CONDITIONS

- Status-post femoral-popliteal bypass

COEXISTING CONDITIONS

- Peripheral vascular disease

LIFESTYLE

- CPA

COMMUNICATION

- English

DISABILITY

- Decreased mobility

SOCIOECONOMIC STATUS

- Middle

SPIRITUAL/RELIGIOUS

- Lutheran

PHARMACOLOGIC

- Ticarcillin disodium/clavulanate potassium (Timentin)

PSYCHOSOCIAL

- Anxiety
- Depression

LEGAL

ETHICAL

ALTERNATIVE THERAPY

PRIORITIZATION

- Antibiotic therapy
- Promote wound healing

DELEGATION

- RN
- Client education

THE MUSCULOSKELETAL AND REPRODUCTIVE SYSTEMS

Level of difficulty: Easy

Overview: This case involves assessment of the client's present problems. The nurse must be knowledgeable about osteomyelitis and the need for immediate medical and nursing interventions to prevent systemic complications and chronic osteomyelitis. The case involves pain management and antibiotic administration with knowledge of unintended effects of analgesic and antibiotic medications, and interventions for these effects.

Client Profile

Mr. Y is a 64-year-old certified public accountant who was discharged from the hospital three weeks ago after amputation of the left great toe related to complete loss of circulation in his extremity. Mr. Y is married and has a 28-year-old daughter in college. His wife is an elementary school teacher. He and his family own a three-bedroom co-op in a newly developed neighborhood.

Case Study

Mr. Y's past medical history includes hypertension and arterial insufficiency. He is status-post (S/P) femoral-popliteal bypass three weeks ago. His family history includes diabetes mellitus (mother) and hypertension and peripheral vascular disease (father). Mr. Y reports that both he and his wife have good health insurance and that he receives a salary while recuperating from surgery. However, he says he is concerned about the continuation of his salary, which is dependent on the length of time the infection will take to heal. Vital signs are:

Blood pressure: 140/94

Pulse: 94

Respirations: 20

Temperature: 101.4° F

The entire foot is tender and warm to touch. There is a moderate amount of mildly odorous drainage coming from the wound. The nursing history and physical examination is completed by the nurse, after which the health care provider reviews the data, asks the client about history of allergies, which the client denies. The health care provider continues the history and physical examination, and a specimen from the infected site is sent to the lab for analysis. The following diagnostic studies are ordered: radionuclide bone scan of the left foot, and a magnetic resonance imaging (MRI), blood culture and gram stain, culture and sensitivity of the wound, white blood cell (WBC) count with differential, and erythrocyte sedimentation rate (ESR). The bone scan reveals infection of the bone marrow, and the MRI identifies calcification of the bones of the foot and provides definitive diagnosis for osteomyelitis. The blood culture and gram stain are positive for P. aeruginosa and Staphylococcus aeruginosa. WBC with differential reveals:

White blood cell (WBC) count: 13,000/mm^3

Neutrophils: 82%

Eosinophils: 4%

Basophils: 2%

Lymphocytes: 43%

Monocytes: 8%

Erythrocyte sedimentation rate (ESR): elevated, 90%

After the multidisciplinary team reviews the diagnostic studies, a diagnosis of osteomyelitis of the left foot is confirmed; the findings are discussed with the client; and plans for surgical debridement are decided upon by the team and Mr. Y. The debridement is done and the surgical plan is to implement high doses of parenteral antibiotics initially followed by oral antibiotics and serial bone scans. Specific orders are written for the surgical team to change the wound dressing during daily rounds.

The following are prescribed:

- Ticarcillin disodium/clavulanate potassium (Timentin) 3.1 g IV q4h
- 0.9% NaCL at 100 mL per hour
- Vitamin A (Aquasol A) 15,000 IU daily
- Vitamin C (ascorbic acid) 500 mg PO two times per day
- ESR, hemoglobin, WBC, albumin levels

Questions

1. Discuss the pathophysiology of osteomyelitis.

2. Discuss groups of persons in whom osteomyelitis is most difficult to manage.

3. Discuss indirect and direct osteomyelitis.

4. Discuss the organism that is the most common cause of osteomyelitis.

5. Discuss the psychosocial impact of the client's amputation on his well-being and the risk that further surgery may be necessary.

6. Discuss common nursing diagnoses for clients with osteomyelitis.

7. What are the purposes for the prescribed orders?

8. What are the most common adverse reactions, drug-to-drug, drug-to-food/herbal interactions for the prescribed medications?

9. Discuss discharge instructions for the client with osteomyelitis.

Osteoarthritis

GENDER

F

AGE

58

SETTING

- Community health clinic

ETHNICITY/CULTURE

- Black American

PREEXISTING CONDITIONS

- Post menopause
- Lack of exercise

COEXISTING CONDITIONS

- Father has severe OA of the hands

LIFESTYLE

- Laundromat manager

COMMUNICATION

DISABILITY

SOCIOECONOMIC STATUS

- Low

SPIRITUAL/RELIGIOUS

- Baptist

PHARMACOLOGIC

- Aspirin (acetylsalicylic acid)
- Antacid (TUMS)
- Celecoxib (Celebrex)
- Calcium carbonate (Os-Cal)
- Capsaicin (Zostrix)

PSYCHOSOCIAL

- Mood changes
- Difficulty adjusting to limitation of use of hands

LEGAL

ETHICAL

- Client should have the right to use alternative therapy with prescribed medications.

ALTERNATIVE THERAPY

- Vegan diet
- Ginseng
- Cayenne pepper

PRIORITIZATION

- Pain management

DELEGATION

- RN
- LPN
- Client education

THE MUSCULOSKELETAL AND REPRODUCTIVE SYSTEMS

Level of difficulty: Moderate

Overview: This case involves a thorough assessment of the client's condition and current over-the-counter and herbal medications. It involves careful inspection and palpation of joints for symmetry, size, shape, color, appearance, and pain, and the use of arthritis disability and discomfort scales to assess the client's functional level for the past week to help determine assistance needed for activities of daily living (ADL). The licensed practical nurse (LPN) can reinforce teaching, after the registered nurse (RN) has initiated it, and continue with assessment procedures.

Client Profile

Ms. C is a 58-year-old female who is seen at the community health clinic for routine annual evaluation. Ms. C is 5′5″ and weighs 150 pounds. The LPN is assigned to take her vital signs, which are:

Blood pressure: 140/84

Pulse: 84

Respirations: 18

Temperature: 98.6° F

Case Study

On initial interview by an RN, Ms. C reports increase in dull, aching pain around the joints of the digits of both hands. Observation of the hands finds evidence of early manifestations of Heberden's and Bouchard's nodes. On further assessment, she reports the use of aspirin to help relieve pain, and antacids (TUMS), to decrease the discomfort in her stomach, which she believes is due to the constant use of aspirin. Continued gathering of data reveals lack of exercise and years of "vegan" diet, but the use of herbs and nuts as supplements. After the RN completes the history and physical, Ms. C is seen by a nurse practitioner (NP) who corroborates data gathered by the nurse, discusses the findings with Ms. C, then orders serum labs to help confirm the presenting symptoms and subjective data. Serum labs are ordered and reveal:

White blood cell (WBC) count: 10,0000 mm^3

Red blood cell (RBC) count: 4.5 million/mm^3

Hemoglobin (Hgb): 13 g/dL

Hematocrit (Hct): 38%

Platelet count (PLT): 250,000 cells/mm^3

Calcium: 8.4 mg/dL

Sodium (Na): 135 mEq/L

Potassium (K+): 4.4 mEq/L

Rheumatoid factor, antinuclear antibody, and erythrocyte sedimentation rate (ESR) are elevated. The labs are reviewed and the client is referred to the community hospital for a magnetic resonance imaging (MRI) of the hands and spine. Ms. C is to return home and have the diagnostic test completed as scheduled, and to continue with follow-up care at the clinic. Ms. C undergoes MRI of the hands and spine, which reveals degenerative changes, especially in the spine. The health care provider discusses the laboratory findings and the result of the MRI with Ms. C, and a diagnosis of osteoarthritis (OA) is confirmed. The health care provider discusses the plan of care for OA, and the following medications are prescribed for her: aspirin (acetylsalicylic acid), topical capsaicin (Zostrix), celecoxib (Celebrex), and calcium (Os-Cal). Ms. C is seen by an RN in the clinic who reviews the prescribed medications with her and allows her to ask questions pertaining to the plan of care as discussed by the health care provider. After dialogue between the client and nurse, Ms. C informs the nurse that she will fill the prescriptions at a pharmacy in her community. A follow-up clinic appointment is scheduled for her, and she leaves the clinic.

The following are prescribed:

- Aspirin (acetylsalicylic acid) 1 g PO three times per day
- Capsaicin (Zostrix) apply to affected areas three to four times per day only
- Celecoxib (Celebrex) 200 mg PO two times per day
- Calcium carbonate (Os-Cal) 1 g PO in the morning and at bedtime

Questions

1. What is your understanding of the above situation?

2. What are some women's health considerations for OA?

3. What is the significance of Heberden's and Bouchard's nodes and their relationship with OA?

4. What are common nursing diagnoses for the client with OA?

5. Discuss nonpharmacologic measures that can be used for clients with OA.

6. What is the role of the physical therapist for clients with OA?

7. What are the purposes for the prescribed medications?

8. What are the most common adverse reactions of the prescribed medications?

9. Discuss the drug-to-drug and drug-to-food/herbal interactions for the prescribed medications.

10. Design a specific pain management plan for the client with OA.

11. What specific information should a nurse provide the client who is discharged to home about topical capsaicin?

CASE STUDY 5

Breast Cancer

GENDER

F

AGE

40

SETTING

- Hospital

ETHNICITY/CULTURE

- Black American

PREEXISTING CONDITIONS

COEXISTING CONDITIONS

- Abscess of the left breast at age 16
- Mother and brother died of breast cancer

LIFESTYLE

- Elementary school teacher
- Uses oral contraceptives

COMMUNICATION

DISABILITY

SOCIOECONOMIC STATUS

- Middle income, but may need supplemental financial support

SPIRITUAL/RELIGIOUS

- Baptist

PHARMACOLOGIC

- Doxorubicin HcL (Adriamycin)
- Cyclophosphamide (Cytoxan)
- Docetaxel (Taxotere)
- Tamoxifen citrate (Nolvadex)
- Ondansetron HcL (Zofran)

PSYCHOSOCIAL

- Anxiety
- Denial
- Fear

LEGAL

ETHICAL

- The client has the right to choose treatment. Is the family able to cope with the present stressors?

ALTERNATIVE THERAPY

- Prayer
- Herbal medications

PRIORITIZATION

- Careful and accurate breast history interview
- Active listening

DELEGATION

- Advanced practice nurse for clinical breast examination
- Client education

THE MUSCULOSKELETAL AND REPRODUCTIVE SYSTEMS

Level of difficulty: Difficult

Overview: This case involves a thorough assessment of the client's condition, including past medical history, family history of cancer including breast cancer, past surgical history, prescribed medications, and herbal supplements the client is currently taking. It requires empathy and the ability to identify with the client's feelings.

Client Profile

Mrs. W is a 40-year-old married client who is seen in the doctor's office for routine examination because she felt a lump in the upper outer quadrant of her left breast during breast self-examination (BSE). Mrs. W is 5′9″ and weighs 194 pounds. During a thorough breast examination, a painless mass that is hard, irregular in shape, and nonmobile in the upper outer quadrant is detected by the health care provider. Her reproductive history reveals one child, age seven years. She reports that her menstrual cycle began at the age of 12. She had used oral contraceptives for several years before her child was conceived. Mrs. W also reports a breast biopsy at the age of 16 for an abscess of the left breast. Her family history includes her mother and a brother who died of breast cancer. Her father, who is 90 years old, and her older sister, who is 42 years old, are both well.

Case Study

Mrs. W is referred for mammography at the community hospital. The mammography is done and reviewed by a radiologist. Mrs. W is later seen by her primary health care provider at his office. The results are discussed, and she is scheduled for diagnostic studies (ultrasound of the left breast and Tru-Cut Core breast biopsy) at a hospital that specializes in oncology. Mrs. W leaves the health care provider's office concerned because of her family history of breast cancer. The diagnostic studies are done and confirm the diagnosis of early stage II cancer of the left breast. Mrs. W is seen by her primary health care provider and an oncologist who discuss her plan of treatment, which will include administration of medication at the hospital and also at home. Mrs. W is admitted to the hospital for treatment for breast cancer and is informed that she will be discharged to home on Tamoxifen citrate (Nolvadex). Her vitals are:

Blood pressure: 134/84

Pulse: 86

Respirations: 18

Temperature: 98.4° F

The following are prescribed:

- Doxorubicin HcL (Adriamycin) 30 mg/m^2 IV for four cycles
- After the four cycles of doxorubicin, start cyclophosphamide (Cytoxan) 4 mg/kg IV over seven days
- Ondansetron HcL (Zofran) 24 mg PO 30 minutes before cyclophosphamide therapy
- Premedicate client with dexamethasone (Decadron) 8 mg two times per day × five days, starting one day prior to docetaxel (Taxotere)

Questions

1. Discuss the various histopathologic types of breast cancer.

2. Discuss etiologies for breast cancer.

3. Discuss cultural and ethnic considerations for breast cancer.

4. Discuss clinical manifestations for breast cancer.

5. Discuss diagnostic studies used to confirm breast cancer.

6. Discuss common nursing diagnoses for breast cancer.

7. What are the purposes for the prescribed medications?

8. What are the most common adverse reactions, drug-to-drug, drug-to-food/herbal interactions of the prescribed medications?

9. Discuss common sites of breast cancer recurrence and metastasis.

10. Discuss client education for breast cancer.

Myasthenia Gravis

GENDER

M

AGE

30

SETTING

- Hospital

ETHNICITY/CULTURE

- Black American

PREEXISTING CONDITIONS

COEXISTING CONDITIONS

- Respiratory tract infection
- Emotional stress

LIFESTYLE

- Law school student
- Lives with parents

COMMUNICATION

DISABILITY

- Activity intolerance related to muscle weakness and fatigue

SOCIOECONOMIC STATUS

- Low

SPIRITUAL/RELIGIOUS

- Baptist

PHARMACOLOGIC

- Pyridostigmine (Mestinon)
- Prednisone (Deltasone)
- Azathioprine (Imuran)

PSYCHOSOCIAL

- Anxiety
- Depression

LEGAL

- Financial support, depending on extent of medical interventions

ETHICAL

ALTERNATIVE THERAPY

PRIORITIZATION

- Airway patency
- Aspiration precaution

DELEGATION

- RN
- Client education

THE MUSCULOSKELETAL AND REPRODUCTIVE SYSTEMS

Level of difficulty: Difficult

Overview: This case involves a thorough assessment of the client's condition with specific focus on complaints of fatigability. It involves current exposure to infectious agents or current infectious problems. The nurse must use critical-thinking skills to prioritize care for the client in a busy emergency department (ED). Questions pertaining to medications and herbal supplements should be a significant part of the history that is taken.

DIFFICULT

Client Profile   **Mr. T** is a 30-year-old law student living at home with his parents. He is expected to graduate at the end of the current semester. Prior to entry into the ED, Mr. T reports having been on amoxicillin as prescribed by his primary health care provider for respiratory infections three weeks ago. Mr. T returned to college after completing the course of amoxicillin but reports feeling unusually tired and was easily fatigued after a two-hour lecture class.

Case Study   In the ED, Mr. T complains of muscle weakness of the eyes and eyelids, has difficulty speaking, and reports noticing that chewing and swallowing were difficult but nonspecific during break period at 10:00 AM. The ED health care provider is notified and immediately responds to the triage nurse's report. Vital signs are:

Blood pressure: 120/80

Pulse: 78

Respirations: 16

Temperature 98.4° F

History and physical are done and find ptosis (drooping of the eyelids) and weakness of facial muscles. Normal pupillary responses to light and accommodation are present. The following diagnostic tests are ordered: serum T_3, T_4, serum protein electrophoresis, and acetylcholine receptor antibodies (AChR) level. The results of the tests reveal: T_3: 205 ng/dL, T_4: 15 ug/dL, serum protein electrophoresis is negative for rheumatoid arthritis, systemic lupus erythematosus and polymyositis, and the AChR level is elevated (1.2 mmol/L). The findings are discussed with Mr. T and his parents as per his approval, and myasthenia gravis (MG) is diagnosed. Mr. T will be discharged to home in 48 hours. He and his parents are involved in an interdisciplinary team discussion before discharge: speech-language pathologist in collaboration with the primary RN, a registered dietitian, and an occupational therapist. The client will return to the clinic in two weeks for reevaluation of medication regimen.

The following are prescribed:

- Pyridostigmine (Mestinon) 60 mg PO daily
- Prednisone (Deltasone) 2 mg/kg/day × one week
- Azathioprine (Imuran) 1 mg/kg/day as maintenance dose

Questions

1. Discuss the incidence and pathophysiology of MG.

2. Discuss clinical manifestations of MG.

3. Discuss assessment and diagnostic findings of MG.

4. Discuss complications of MG.

5. Discuss the differences in care of the client with myasthenic crisis and cholinergic crisis.

6. Discuss plasmapheresis and its relationship to MG.

7. Discuss surgical management of MG.

8. What are the purposes for the prescribed medications?

9. What are the most common adverse reactions, drug-to-drug, drug-to-food/herbal interactions of the prescribed medications?

10. Discuss client education for MG.

Index

Notes

Notes

Notes

Notes

Notes

Notes

Notes

Notes

Notes

Notes

Notes

Notes